SpringerBriefs in Applied Sciences and Technology

Computational Intelligence

Series Editor

Janusz Kacprzyk, Systems Research Institute, Polish Academy of Sciences, Warsaw, Poland

SpringerBriefs in Computational Intelligence are a series of slim high-quality publications encompassing the entire spectrum of Computational Intelligence. Featuring compact volumes of 50 to 125 pages (approximately 20,000-45,000 words), Briefs are shorter than a conventional book but longer than a journal article. Thus Briefs serve as timely, concise tools for students, researchers, and professionals.

Rahul Saxena · Mahipal Jadeja · Vikrant Bhateja

Exploring Susceptible-Infectious-Recovered (SIR) Model for COVID-19 Investigation

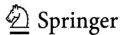
Springer

Rahul Saxena
Department of Computer Science
and Engineering
Malaviya National Institute of Technology
Jaipur
Jaipur, Rajasthan, India

Department of Information Technology
Manipal University Jaipur
Jaipur, Rajasthan, India

Vikrant Bhateja
Department of Electronics
and Communication Engineering
Shri Ramswaroop Memorial College
of Engineering and Management
(SRMCEM)
Lucknow, Uttar Pradesh, India

Dr. A.P.J. Abdul Kalam Technical
University
Lucknow, Uttar Pradesh, India

Mahipal Jadeja
Department of Computer Science
and Engineering
Malaviya National Institute of Technology
Jaipur
Jaipur, Rajasthan, India

ISSN 2191-530X   ISSN 2191-5318 (electronic)
SpringerBriefs in Applied Sciences and Technology
ISSN 2625-3704   ISSN 2625-3712 (electronic)
SpringerBriefs in Computational Intelligence
ISBN 978-981-19-4174-0   ISBN 978-981-19-4175-7 (eBook)
https://doi.org/10.1007/978-981-19-4175-7

This Springer imprint is published by the registered company Springer Nature Singapore Pte Ltd.
The registered company address is: 152 Beach Road, #21-01/04 Gateway East, Singapore 189721, Singapore

Preface

The book encompasses various aspects of the Covid-19 disease spread pattern and a comparative analysis with a few other disease models of the past. The objective is to understand the basic SIR model characteristics and how it conforms to the real-time data to validate a few facts regarding the rise and fall parameters of the growth rate of the infection. More importantly, experimental results over real-time data conform to the theory and the deviations. The model dynamics-based severity comparison of the two spread waves of Covid-19 in two consecutive years with respect to the model parameters is also highlighted in the book. The book also discusses the comparison of lockdown periods of both the waves.

The flow of the book is organized as follows: Chap. 1 provides a general introduction to the COVID-19, its impact, and effects and highlights the need to understand the mathematical modelling of the disease. Chapter 2 reviews the state-of-the-art work of various epidemic models for various outbreaks. It further presents a description of the SIR model and its mathematical setup. Chapter 3 analyses the basic growth pattern and spread pattern of the Covid-19 disease. Chapter 4 shows how SIR modelling parameters fit to the growth model and how varying the model parameters can affect the epidemic spread followed by an investigative analysis and its implications. Chapter 5 presents the analysis of the obtained results. Chapter 6 presents insights into the second wave of COVID-19 using SIR modelling based on change(s) in the parametric values of the model as discussed in Chaps. 4 and 5. Finally, Chap. 7 concludes the book.

Jaipur, India   Rahul Saxena
Jaipur, India   Mahipal Jadeja
Lucknow, India   Vikrant Bhateja

Acknowledgement

I (Mr. Rahul Saxena) am writing this acknowledgement on the behalf of all the authors of this book.

First of all, I thank the Almighty God, who gave me the opportunity and strength to carry out this work.

Expression of feelings by words makes them less significant when it comes to making a statement of gratitude.

I would like to thank Manipal University Jaipur and Malaviya National Institute of Technology for carrying out this work. The lab, printing, library, etc. facilities of both the institutions have played a significant role in carrying out the experimental work and simulations. Moreover, I am thankful to the official staff of both the institutions for providing the conducive environment which helped a lot to present the study and findings in the form of this book.

I would like to express my deep sense of gratitude to my parents, wife, brother, and other family members who supported me and provided the strength to carry out this work.

Thanks are also due to my friends and colleagues who had provided their valuable advice and knowledge to help me out in my project.

I am also thankful to the previous researchers whose published work has been consulted and cited in the book.

Contents

About the Authors

Mr. Rahul Saxena is currently working as Assistant Professor in the Department of Information technology, Manipal University Jaipur, since 2015, and pursuing Ph.D. from Malaviya National Institute of Technology, Jaipur, since 2019. He completed his Masters from Manipal University Jaipur in the year 2015. He has been awarded with Gold Medal for Excellence in Education in Masters. He completed his B.E. from Birla Institute of Technology, Mesra, in year 2013. His areas of research and interest include social networks analysis, machine learning, graph algorithms, parallel processing, etc. He has several conference, journal articles, and book chapters published in Springer, IEEE, etc. in the related domains of research. Apart from this, he is an active review member in many Scopus indexed journals of Springer, Elsevier, and has served as organizing committee member in various international conferences of IEEE, Springer, in various capacities like Convener, Session chair, TPC, etc.

Dr. Mahipal Jadeja received his Ph.D. degree from Dhirubhai Ambani Institute of Information and Communication Technology (DA-IICT), India, in 2018. He currently works at Malaviya National Institute of Technology (MNIT Jaipur) as an assistant professor. His research interests include theoretical computer science, graph theory, algorithms, social network analysis, and graph neural networks. He has published several journal articles and book chapters in these domains. His research work is presented at reputed international conferences including GSB-SIGIR 2015 (Chile), WAAC 2016 (Japan), and SCAI-ICTIR 2017 (Netherlands). Apart from this, he is an active reviewer for many SCI/Scopus indexed journals. He has served as a TPC member for many conferences including AISE 2020 (Springer international conference).

Dr. Vikrant Bhateja is Associate Professor in the Department of Electronics and Communication Engineering (ECE), Shri Ramswaroop Memorial College of Engineering and Management (SRMCEM), Lucknow (Affiliated to AKTU), and also Dean (Academics) in the same college. He is doctorate in ECE (Bio-Medical Imaging) with a total academic teaching experience of 19 years with around 180 publications in reputed international conferences, journals, and online book chapter contributions; out of which 31 papers are published in SCIE indexed high impact factored journals. Among the international conference publications, four papers have received "Best Paper Award." Among the SCIE publications, one paper published in Review of Scientific Instruments (RSI) Journal (under American International Publishers) has been selected as "Editor Choice Paper of the Issue" in 2016. He has been instrumental in chairing/co-chairing around 25 international conferences in India and abroad as Publication/TPC chair and edited 45 book volumes from Springer-Nature as a corresponding/co-editor/author on date. He has delivered nearly 20 keynotes, invited talks in international conferences, ATAL, TEQIP, and other AICTE sponsored FDPs and STTPs. He is Editor-in-Chief of IGI Global–International Journal of Natural Computing and Research (IJNCR) an ACM and DBLP indexed journal since 2017. He has guest edited special issues in reputed SCIE indexed journals under Springer-Nature and Elsevier. He is Senior Member of IEEE and Life Member of CSI.

Acronyms

COVID-19	2019 novel coronavirus disease
DL	Deep Learning
ML	Machine Learning
SARS	Severe Acute Respiratory Syndrome
SEIR	Susceptible, Exposed, Infected, and Recovered model
SI	Susceptible and Infected model
SIR	Susceptible, Infected, and Recovered model
SIS	Susceptible, Infected, and Susceptible model
WHO	World Health Organization
ZIKF	Zika Virus Fever

Chapter 1
Introduction

According to WHO [2], the novel Coronavirus (Covid-19) epidemic began in Wuhan, China, on the 2nd of January, 2020, and was declared a Public Health Emergency of International Concern (PHEIC) on the 30th of January, 2020. According to the same research in [2], the WHO designated this ailment coronavirus disease (Covid-19) in February 2020. The number of Corona-positive patients has climbed to 4.53 million, resulting in 307 thousand deaths, as of May 16th, 2020. The disease was spreading so swiftly that it had resulted in $1,484,287$ Corona-positive cases and $88,507$ fatalities in the United States; $2,76,505$ positive cases and $27,563$ deaths in Spain; $2,24,760$ positive cases and $31,763$ deaths in Italy; and so on in many other countries [3]. With a total of more than $86,000$ positive patients, India had overcome China and ranks 11th in the list of countries (as of 16th May) with the most positive patients. The pandemic has a deep impact because of the disease's high infectious nature, which spreads at an exponential rate through contractual transmission, largely through body contact (through hands or any other body parts). The trauma is still occurring, and given the current rate of expansion and conditions, it is expected to worsen in some locations. Governments of respective countries seek insights from doctors, scientists, and economists to prepare strategies for dealing with the current situation. Since the category of this infectious virus is fairly new, there is a lack of knowledge about its spread patterns and dynamics, its growth cause, building mechanism etc. Many studies and research are being conducted worldwide to identify vital information about the various aspects of the disease. But this evolving nature both of the disease and its effects makes it very hard to make strategic policies in synchrony with time. By the time the decisions of lockdowns along with travel restrictions (both national and international) were implemented, the spread had already burst out to a greater extent. Even countries that are following strict social distancing measures are struggling to contain the growth burst. The book discusses about these aspects in detail and feels that this is the only way out, given the current information about the virus to counter it. The next section, thus, discusses the impacts of Covid-19 on various countries briefly.

1.1   Worldwide Impacts of Covid-19

All of this raises concerns about how the virus has wreaked havoc on countries' economies and diverse sectors of growth. Given in the context of India, the GDP downfall chart is as per [4]. Due to the COVID-19 epidemic, GDP growth is expected to dip from 5.7% to 5.2% in the fiscal year 2021, according to domestic rating agency Crisis [4]. According to it, it's a big major threat than the 2008 global financial crisis as it not only impacts the economic activities and financial stability but also brings with it enormous human sufferings, not witnessed in decades. Another agency named Standard & Poors (S & P) has given a revised estimation of the growth figures after the pandemic invasion which shows a significant drop in the values estimated earlier.

A similar economic disruption in other countries, such as the United States, Italy, China, and Spain, is possible, as reported by the BBC on its homepage [1]. This means a heavy economic loss pertaining not only to a single nation but on a world stage which hurts even more. Moreover, a lot of precious human lives are lost and still many will die at the hands of this virus which is sadistic and turns to be a harsh reality and will be remembered as a black past. Many attempts from the medical science community worldwide are on to find the cure for this disease which includes some recent state-of-the-art research in the field of computer vision [5] citesingh2022contrast [6]. The Times of India report shows the medical fraternity of various countries that are making trials and attempts to develop drugs that can provide an answer to the queries raised by this heath-endangered virus but it seems that the world has to wait for quite a some time to have this cure at their hand.

Because the treatment for Covid-19 is unknown at this time, people must exercise caution and foresight in dealing with the problem. To combat this epidemic, one must first comprehend the virus's spread pattern. This will offer a new notion of how to do a prediction analysis of the disease's progress so that various policies and strategic decisions can be framed. This includes how long the pandemic will be on a higher curve, what is the expected time after which the growth is expected to decline, what are the factors that can be controlled to increase the recovery rate and bring down the infection growth rate, etc. Answers to all these questions help in planning for maintaining stocks of basic needs and determining the capacity of medical health equipment, kits, and other facilities, so that if needed, these facilities can be increased timely. Understanding spread patterns and dynamics helps in having a futuristic view. In order to answer the above-mentioned questions, mathematical modelling can be applied. Therefore, the next section discusses the SIR model.

1.2   SIR Model: A Good Fit for Modelling Covid-19

SIR model was created by Ronald Ross [7] to explain the growth pattern and malaria life. Since then, it has served as a conceptual paradigm for explaining the spread of many viral illnesses. This book examines the concept and operation of this basic model using data from a few Indian states to see how the disease's transmission pattern matches Ross' mathematical model. The book attempts to figure out how Covid-19 modelling differs as compared to other epidemic illness models that use the same SIR model.

For a better understanding of the mathematical modelling, results are simulated for four regions of India: Rajasthan, Gujarat, Maharashtra, and Delhi, where the pandemic strike is severe. The initial growth trend study (conducted over the data from the point of time of the first infected case found in any of the regions till 12th July 2020) showed that the rate at which the infection is propagating follows a logistic regression curve. The curve fits accurately to the actual trend of growth with R^2 value of more than 99%. The curve fitting accounts for such high accuracy as the infection is on a rise in India till date and follows almost an exponential trajectory. However, it has been demonstrated that the model has limitations and cannot be used to do trend analysis as a generic prediction model. Further, other vital and key information insights cannot be derived from it. To overcome these limitations, the most used Susceptible-Infected-Recovery (SIR) epidemic model is explored which offers more profound mathematics to model the pandemic. Considering the global reproduction number value $R_0 = 6.0$ for the Coronavirus, it has been shown how the current data values (for Indian states) fit to the model. Based on this, further, the effect of lockdown in the four regions of India has been analysed and how lockdown has helped to reduce the effective contact rate has been verified. With respect to this SIR model-based growth rate evaluation, the severity of Covid-19 with other epidemics like SARs, Ebola, Measles, Nipah, Influenza, and MERS has been compared. Further exploring the model dynamics in detail, some interesting results like up to how many maximum individuals in a particular region can get infected, how long the pandemic will prevail, etc. have been derived. The book also presents an interesting viewpoint from the futuristic perspective of determining the number of individuals to be vaccinated depending upon the herd immunity. Since the model has a set of assumptions associated with it, mainly due to evolving data and other factors like change in contact rate, virus evolution, etc., predictions based on the mathematical structure developed may seem far from reality, but still offers realistic perspectives on near-term trends and outcome inclination.

1.3   Organization of the Book

The overall organization of the book is as follows: This chapter covers the disease, its impact and effects on the countries, and the necessity to understand its mathematical modelling. In **Chap.** 2, the SIR model and its mathematical setup are briefly discussed. The chapter also discusses state-of-the-art epidemic models for various outbreaks. In **Chap.** 3, the growth trend of Covid-19 is analysed with the help of a logistic regression model for three Indian states and an union territory. The growing pattern of infection dissemination data is closely matched by the logistic curve. However, after reviewing the data, it is determined that a more robust model is required. How SIR parameters fit into the growth model is shown in **Chap.** 4 and also how changing model parameters can help for a better understanding of epidemic control. As a result of the model parameters, a little investigation is carried out to visualize the decline in the contact rate during the lockdown period in India. In Chap. 5, the results and discussion of an experimental investigation using real data and model postulates are presented. The findings are described and interpreted in further detail in the same chapter. **Chapter** 6 presents a detailed exploration of the SIR model for the second wave of Covid-19, and a comprehensive comparison of the dynamics of the disease with the first wave is done. Finally, **Conclusion** section wraps up the major findings and analysis.

References

1. BBC news Homepage: https://www.bbc.com/news/business-51706225. Accessed on 24/03/2022
2. Coronavirus (COVID-19) outbreak, WHO Homepage: https://www.who.int/westernpacific/emergencies/covid-19, Accessed on 24/03/2022
3. WorldOmeter Homepage: https://www.worldometers.info/coronavirus/, Accessed on 24/03/2022
4. Quartz India Homepage: https://qz.com/india/1827925/how-will-coronavirus-impact-indias-economy-as-per-moodys-fitch/, Accessed on 24/03/20224
5. Banerjee, A., Bhattacharya, R., Bhateja, V., Kumar Singh, P., Sarkar, R. et al.: Cofe-net: An ensemble strategy for computer-aided detection for covid-19. Measurement, **187**, 110289 (2022)
6. Dikshit, A., Bhateja, V., Rai., A.: Discrete wavelet transform-based fusion of mammogram images for contrast improvement. In: Advances in Micro-Electronics, Embedded Systems and IoT, pp. 203–210. Springer (2022)
7. Dworkin, J., Tan, S.Y.: Ronald ross (1857–1932): discoverer of malaria's life cycle. Singapore Med. J. **52**(7), 466–467 (2011)

Chapter 2
Epidemic Studies and Mathematical Setup of SIR Model

This chapter deals with a brief overview of the epidemic modelling of various viral spreads. The chapter discusses the prediction and trend analysis mechanisms using Machine Learning (ML), statistical, and Deep Learning (DL) approaches. The chapter further discusses the mathematical formulations and structure of SIR epidemic modelling. The model is described in terms of summation of three dependent quantities: *Number of Susceptibles*, *Number of Infected people*, and *Number of people recovered* from the disease. Further, this simple linear equation is expanded in terms of three nonlinear differential equations which are solved to find the estimates and perform the result analysis.

2.1 Epidemic Studies and Modelling: The State-of-the-Art Techniques

Epidemic modelling has been an area of great interest and many academicians and researchers in the past have laid down important theories and postulates related to it. The SI (Susceptible-Infected) and SIR (Susceptible-Infected-Recovered) models of epidemic modelling were first established by Sir Ronald Ross et al. [2] to reproduce the transmission mechanism of malarial infection. Three basic nonlinear ordinary differential equations with no explicit formula solution make up the model. Since then, many versions of this basic model have been developed by loosening certain assumptions and/or adding more factors to study. For diseases that endure for long periods of time, such as $10-20$ years, Hethcote et al. [9] investigated three mathematical models: Susceptible-Infected (SI), SIR with non-dynamic vitality, and SIR with dynamic vitality epidemic models. To repeat the cycle, the model incorporates the birth and regeneration of susceptibles. Anderson et al. [3] provided their viewpoint

R. Saxena et al., *Exploring Susceptible-Infectious-Recovered (SIR) Model for COVID-19 Investigation*, SpringerBriefs in Computational Intelligence, https://doi.org/10.1007/978-981-19-4175-7_2

on stochastic epidemic models and the statistical analysis that goes with them. The authors looked into a number of epidemic modelling topics including modelling an infectious disease's demand on adjacent sick people, vaccination, and herd immunity. The work brought up other lines of inquiry into the proposed epidemic modelling under conditions of longevity, rapid rate spread, and so on. The SIR model was used by Berge et al. [5] to try to explain the spread pattern of the 2013 *Ebola* pandemic in Africa. The endemic equilibrium model was described, which states that the infection dies when the vulnerable population is depleted.

Rachah et al. [18] analysed the Ebola outbreak using the SEIR model, which is a variant of the standard SIR model with one more state exposed included in. The authors backed up the model's conclusions by assigning real-world values to the model parameters. The acquired results were in agreement with the SEIR model's theorems and lemmas. Based on the findings, the scientists devised an optimal vaccination-based control plan for Ebola. Another SEIR model-based investigation on Ebola was conducted by Sylvie et al. [8]. The model was based on seven compartments: susceptible, exposed, infected asymptomatic, infected symptomatic, hospitalized, recovered, and deceased people. Because the model divided the urban and rural populations, epidemic management measures differed as a result of increased awareness through educational efforts, vaccination, and other means. In a research study published in Nature, Kato et al. [12] illustrated how both preventive and confinement measures are required to curb viral spread using the SIR model propositions.

Mkhatshwa et al. [15] evaluated the model parameter values for the *SARS* outbreak over the real data for the disease and then compared the results to the prior submissions over the same disease. In November 2015, Mpshe et al. [16] reported on a SIR model-based analysis of the *Zika* virus fever (ZIKVF) outbreak in Cape Verde. The model calculated the virus's R_0 value and investigated the components' respective effects on R_0. The researchers discovered that increasing the death rate of *Aedes mosquitoes* and the pace of patient recovery can help reduce epidemics. Riou et al. [19] did a comparison analysis utilizing model-estimated values for *ZIKV* and *Chikenghunia virus*. The study compared the pace of infection spread, as well as other parameters such as temperature and humidity, to examine important differences in the behavioural pattern of the two diseases. Sultana et al. [22] and Biswas et al. [6] used the SIR model to analyse the lethal Nipah viral catastrophe in Bangladesh (which prevailed continuously from 2001 to 2014, with the mortality rate being 76%). Xian-Xian Liu et al. [13] proposed the SEAIRD prediction model. The development and control of epidemics are related to model and forecast patterns, and epidemic control is projected as a continually changing process. The results of this modified model are contrasted with the predictions of the traditional SEIR model for the Covid-19 outbreak in the United States.

The forecast findings from the adaptive SEAIRD model for the Covid-19 epidemic data in the United States are demonstrated to align well with the actual pandemic curve. Shinde et al. [21] published a recent valuation on the trend prediction of Covid-19. The methods were divided into four categories by the authors of the paper: (i) access to large datasets from WHO/national agencies [23] and [20]; (ii) data from social media; (iii) stochastic and mathematical models [14, 24, 25]; (iv) data science and machine learning models [4, 10, 11]. The authors found, however, that data trend analysis is dependent on a variety of circumstances and that there is no single method or technique for all the cases for predictions. Machine learning/data science models such as logistic regression, Weibull equation, and others were found to be effective in predicting infection spread trend analysis forecasts. They also considered the effects of illness on people of all ages and genders, as well as quarantine measures and initiatives for better disease management. The significance of these models, on the other hand, is limited to infection growth rate prediction. As a result, mathematical models simulating epidemic dynamics appear to have a better chance of succeeding.

Most mathematical epidemic models developed for the study of infectious outbreaks, such as SIER, SIERS, and others, are based on the core SIR model and its variations, such as SIER, SIERS, and others, as described above. There are some stochastic technique-based mathematical models for analysing epidemics and their effects. However, the fundamental SIR model is mostly used in the literature to predict and analyse epidemics of other forms of contagions such as SARS, Malaria, EBOLA, Swine Flu, and others. Using the insights learned from the previous models, [7, 17], a similar estimation-based model has been investigated for Covid-19 spread out in this book using real-time data. For four of India's most severely affected locations, the growth pattern of infection, recovery rate, and death rate were examined. The model parameters were estimated based on the information supplied. With the use of parameter values (taken from the literature) and the same underlying SIR model, a full comparison of Covid-19 with other disorders has also been drawn. This allows us to forecast the direction of the trend in the future. Preventive measures (such as health-care arrangements, quarantine measures, social isolation, and so on) can also be planned ahead of time. The vaccination process is also considered for gaining a sense of what future action should be taken with respect to the prevention of the disease. Table 2.1 presents a summarized overview of a few prominent state-of-the-art works discussed so far.

2.2 SIR Mathematical Modelling

The state-of-the-art discussions differentiate *epidemic* and *pandemic* burst out as follows:

- The outburst of the disease to a mass in a very short period of time is referred to as *epidemic*.
- When an epidemic spreads across the globe, it is referred to as *pandemic*.

The covid-19 outbreak has spread venomously across the globe due to which approximately 180 countries have been hit badly across the globe till date. The disease has a very high spread rate and can affect as many as 5–6 people out of 10 from a single infected patient. The spread of any contagious disease depends upon two factors: the amount of contact between the persons and the chance that an

Table 2.1 Few prominent state-of-the-art contributions and study for epidemic spread

Article title	Authors	Year	Findings
Modelling approach to investigate the dynamics of Zika virus fever: A neglected disease in Africa	Mpeshe, Saul C and Nyerere, Nkuba and Sanga, Stephano	2017	Presented SIR model-based analysis of the *Zika* virus fever (ZIKVF) outbreak in Cape Verde. The model calculated the virus's R_0 value and investigated the components' respective effects on R_0. The researchers discovered that increasing the death rate of *Aedes mosquitoes* and the pace of patient recovery can help reduce epidemics
A comparative analysis of Chikungunya and Zika transmission	Riou, Julien and Poletto, Chiara and Boëlle, Pierre-Yves	2017	Did a comparison analysis utilizing model-estimated values for *ZIKV* and *Chikenghunia virus*. The study compared the pace of infection spread, as well as other parameters such as temperature and humidity, to examine important differences in the behavioural pattern of the two diseases
Analysis, simulation, and optimal control of a SEIR model for Ebola virus with demographic effects	Rachah, Amira and Torres, Delfim FM	2017	Analysed the Ebola outbreak using the SEIR model, which is a variant of the standard SIR model with one more state exposed included in. The authors backed up the model's conclusions by assigning real-world values to the model parameters. The acquired results were in agreement with the SEIR model's theorems and lemmas
Forecasting models for coronavirus disease (COVID-19): a survey of the state of the art	Shinde, Gitanjali R and Kalamkar, Asmita B and Mahalle, Parikshit N and Dey, Nilanjan and Chaki, Jyotismita and Hassanien, Aboul Ella	2020	Presented a study on the prediction of Covid-19 using stochastic, probabilistic, data science, and machine learning-based approaches
A new SEAIRD pandemic prediction model with clinical and epidemiological data analysis on COVID-19 outbreak	Liu, Xian-Xian and Fong, Simon James and Dey, Nilanjan and Crespo, Rubén González and Herrera-Viedma, Enrique	2021	Proposed SEAIRD prediction model in which epidemic control is projected as a continually changing process. The results of this modified model are contrasted with the predictions of the traditional SEIR model for the Covid-19 outbreak in the United States

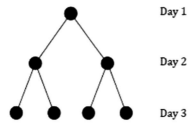

Fig. 2.1 Exponential growth rate of disease

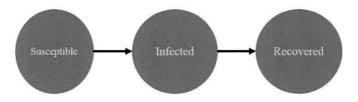

Fig. 2.2 Three stages of SIR Model (S: Susceptible, I: Infected, and R: Recovered) [1]

infected person spreads the disease to the person in contact with him or her. If it is assumed that the transmission probability of disease from an infected person is 1 or 100%, then, if every infected person meets two other persons before being recovered, the disease spread will be rapid. Assuming that if the recovery period for the disease is one day, then it means that the number of sick people will double each day. This spread growth rate will take the shape of an exponential function expressed as

$$I = 2^t - 1 \qquad (2.1)$$

Here, 'I' represents the total number of infected people and 't' is the total time elapsed from the day infection has started. This growth pattern can diagrammatically be represented as (Fig. 2.1).

This simple basic growth model defines an increment in the infected population given the constant multiplication factor. However, the SIR model presents a more realistic approach to model the disease. It takes into account more number of factors and variables. The SIR model has three transition phases: Susceptible, Infected, and Recovered. The model makes an assumption that the infected people once recover from the disease will never again be in the susceptible phase. The cycle of disease moves as per Fig. 2.2. Let the total population in consideration be of size 'N', then relations between the three categories of the population at any time 't' can be defined as

$$S(t) + I(t) + R(t) = N \qquad (2.2)$$

Let the initial values be defined as $S(0) = S_0$, $I(0) = I_0$, and $R(0) = R_0$. Now based upon these variables defined, the task will be to find out the followings: $\frac{ds}{dt} =?$, $\frac{dI}{dt} =?$, and $\frac{dR}{dt} =?$. These are referred to as the rate of change of susceptible, rate of change of infected persons, and rate of change of recovered population, respectively. To evaluate these rate of change values, let's define the susceptible population at time instance '$t + dt$':

$$S(t + dt) = S(t) - aSI.dt \qquad (2.3)$$

Rearranging the terms, we get

$$\frac{S(t+dt)-S(t)}{dt} = -aSI$$

The left-hand side part of the equation corresponds to the definition of derivative or rate of change of susceptible with respect to time which finally can be written as

$$\frac{dS}{dt} = -aSI \qquad (2.4)$$

Equation 2.4 has a proportionality constant 'a' defined as transmission rate. The relationship specifies the conversion of the susceptible population to the infected with a transmission rate 'a'. The negative sign indicates that since the number of susceptible persons are getting converted to infected, the number of susceptible in the complete population is reducing. Thus, there is a negative correlation between variables 'S' and 'I'. Similarly, the rate of change of recovered patients with respect to time can be defined as

$$\frac{dR}{dt} = b.I \qquad (2.5)$$

Here, 'b' stands for the recovery rate factor with which the infected population 'I' recovers. Finally, upon solving, the rate of change of infected population with respect to time can be defined as

$$\frac{dI}{dt} = aSI - bI \qquad (2.6)$$

Equation 2.6 defines the rate at which the number of people is getting infected in time 't'. It is represented as the difference between the number of susceptibles and the number of susceptibles getting infected in time 't'. Further, by exploring these equations in detail, a few interesting facts can be derived.

From Eq. 2.6, initial rate of change can be defined as

$$\frac{dI}{dt_{t=0}} = aS_0b - bI_0 \qquad (2.7)$$

This rate of change must be less than zero. Because if this rate of change of infected person is greater than zero, then the epidemic is likely to spread. Hence, we can derive the condition to prevent the spread of the disease as follows

$$\frac{dI}{dt_{t=0}} < 0 \text{ or } a S_0 - b_0 < 0$$

This implies

$$\frac{a S_0}{b} < 1 \tag{2.8}$$

This factor $\frac{a S_0}{b}$ is defined as the reproduction rate R_0. Based upon these simple nonlinear differential equations, model parameters are built (discussed further in Chap. 4).

References

1. Collins, J., Abdelal, N.: Spread of Disease. https://calculate.org.au/wp-content/uploads/sites/15/2018/10/spread-of-disease.pdf, Accessed on 24/03/2022
2. Anderson., R.M.:Discussion: the kermack-mckendrick epidemic threshold theorem. Bull. Math. Biol. **53**(1–2), 1 (1991)
3. Andersson, H., Britton, T.: Stochastic Epidemic Models and Their Statistical Analysis, vol. 151. Springer Science & Business Media (2012)
4. Batista, M.: Estimation of the final size of the second phase of coronavirus epidemic by the logistic model (2020)
5. Berge, T., Lubuma, JM-S., Moremedi, G.M., Morris, N., Kondera-Shava, R.: A simple mathematical model for Ebola in Africa. J. Biol. Dyn. **11**(1), 42–74 (2017)
6. Ali Biswas, M.H., Haque, M.M., Duvvuru, G.: A mathematical model for understanding the spread of nipah fever epidemic in Bangladesh. In: 2015 International Conference on Industrial Engineering and Operations Management (IEOM), pp. 1–8. IEEE (2015)
7. Cooper, I., Mondal, A., Antonopoulos, C.G.: A sir model assumption for the spread of covid-19 in different communities. Chaos, Solitons & Fractals **139**, 110057 (2020)
8. SYLVIE DIANE DJIOMBA NJANKOU and Farai Nyabadza: An optimal control model for Ebola virus disease. J. Biol. Syst. **24**(01), 29–49 (2016)
9. Hethcote, H.W.: Three basic epidemiological models. In: Applied Mathematical Ecology, pp. 119–144. Springer (1989)
10. Hu, Z., Ge, Q., Li, S., Jin, L., Xiong, M.: Evaluating the effect of public health intervention on the global-wide spread trajectory of covid-19 (2020)
11. Jia, L., Li, K., Jiang, Y., Guo, X. et al.: Prediction and analysis of coronavirus disease 2019 (2020). arXiv:2003.05447
12. Kato, Fuminori, Tainaka, Kei-ichi, Sone, Shogo, Morita, Satoru, Iida, Hiroyuki, Yoshimura, Jin: Combined effects of prevention and quarantine on a breakout in sir model. Sci. Rep. **1**, 10 (2011)
13. Liu, X-X., Fong, S.J., Dey, N., González Crespo, R., Herrera-Viedma, E.: A new seaird pandemic prediction model with clinical and epidemiological data analysis on covid-19 outbreak. Appl. Intel. 1–37 (2021)
14. Magal, P., Webb, G.: Predicting the number of reported and unreported cases for the covid-19 epidemic in South Korea, Italy, France and Germany. Italy, France and Germany (March 19, 2020) (2020)
15. Mkhatshwa, T. Mummert, A.: Modeling super-spreading events for infectious diseases: case study sars (2010). arXiv:1007.0908

16. Mpeshe, S.C., Nyerere, N., Sanga, S.: Modeling approach to investigate the dynamics of zika virus fever: A neglected disease in Africa. Int. J. Adv. Appl. Math. Mech **4**(3), 14–21 (2017)
17. Nesteruk, I.: Estimations of the coronavirus epidemic dynamics in South Korea with the use of sir model. Preprint.] ResearchGate (2020)
18. Rachah, A., Torres, D.F.M.: Analysis, simulation and optimal control of a seir model for ebola virus with demographic effects (2017). arXiv:1705.01079
19. Riou, Julien, Poletto, Chiara, Boëlle, Pierre-Yves.: A comparative analysis of chikungunya and zika transmission. Epidemics **19**, 43–52 (2017)
20. Russo, L., Anastassopoulou, C., Tsakris, A., Bifulco, G.N., Campana, E.F., Toraldo, G., Siettos, C.: Tracing DAY-ZERO forecasting the fade out of the covid-19 outbreak in Lombardy. Italy: a compartmental modelling and numerical optimization approach (2020)
21. Shinde, G.R., Kalamkar, A.B., Mahalle, P.N., Dey, N., Chaki, J., Hassanien, A.E.: Forecasting models for coronavirus disease (covid-19): a survey of the state-of-the-art. SN Comput. Sci. **1**(4), 1–15 (2020)
22. Sultana, J., Podder, C.N. et al.: Mathematical analysis of Nipah virus infections using optimal control theory. J. Appl. Math. Phys. **4**(06), 1099 (2016)
23. Teles, P.: Predicting the evolution of sars-covid-2 in portugal using an adapted sir model previously used in South Korea for the mers outbreak (2020). arXiv:2003.10047
24. Victor, A.: Mathematical predictions for covid-19 as a global pandemic. Available at SSRN 3555879 (2020)
25. Wang, H., Zhang, Y., Lu, S., Wang, S.: Tracking and forecasting milepost moments of the epidemic in the early-outbreak: framework and applications to the covid-19. F1000Research 9 (2020)

Chapter 3
Understanding and Analysing the Spread Pattern of Covid-19

The chapter here defines the exponential trajectory of the growth dynamics of the disease. From infection growth trend to recovery and casualty growth rate, all follow an exponential rise with respect to time. Thus, a logistic model-based fit to make predictions for the disease looks good. However, further exploration of the model for understanding disease dynamics based on the logistic curve is not possible. The chapter finally concludes with the limitations of logistic curve-based analysis of the model and defines the need for exploration of disease based on epidemic mathematical models like SIR.

3.1 Exponential Growth Rate Analysis of Covid-19

The chapter discusses the virus spreading and infection growth mechanism. The chapter also contains parameter behaviour analysis based on SIR modelling. The data of a few regions of India where the viral attack has been predominantly high as compared to other states are considered. The numbers until 12th July 2020 for these states are provided in Table 3.1 based on the information from [3]. The numbers differ in the three metrics for the four states because the infection rate and the recovery rate varied in all the four regions.

For contagion spread and healing rate trend, the curve follows an exponential growth trend. The rate of progression, on the other hand, varies based on a variety of circumstances. Nonetheless, the general curvature follows logistic equation described as

$$y = \frac{a}{1 + e^{-c(x-d)}} + b \tag{3.1}$$

R. Saxena et al., *Exploring Susceptible-Infectious-Recovered (SIR) Model for COVID-19 Investigation*, SpringerBriefs in Computational Intelligence, https://doi.org/10.1007/978-981-19-4175-7_3

Table 3.1 State-wise stats for number of people infected, recovered, and dead till 12th July 2020 [1]

State	First case reported on	Infected cases	Recovered patients	Casualty
Rajasthan	4/3/2020	23748	17869	503
Gujarat	20/3/2020	40941	28649	2032
Maharashtra	9/3/2020	246600	136985	10116
Delhi	2/3/2020	110921	87692	3334

Table 3.2 Parametric values for the logistic fit as per Eq. 3.1

States	Logistic Parameter estimated values			
	a	b	c	d
Rajasthan	8.0991e+04	−1.1698e+03	3.1427e-02	1.5326e+02
Gujarat	1.0757e+05	−4.4275e+03	2.8945e-02	1.2263e+02
Maharashtra	3.4110e+06	−7.5880e+03	3.6533e-02	1.9026e+02
Delhi	2.3187e+05	3.7039e+02	6.4986e-02	1.2802e+02

Equation 3.1 has x representing infected cases until July 12th, 2020, and y represents the logistic function's closest fit to the actual value. Parameter a is the maximum value that can be obtained using the fit, b is the shift in non-horizontal direction, c is the slope, and d is the non-vertical shift from the axis. The initial guess values are $a = 1$, $b = 0$, $c = 1$, and $d = 0$. The equation for the most basic logistic curve is obtained by plugging these numbers into Eq. 3.1:

$$y = \frac{1}{1 + e^{-x}} \tag{3.2}$$

Parameter values for the four different state instances are estimated based on this initial estimation. This estimate is based on the datasets' curve fitting. Table 3.2 displays the estimated parameter values.

Each day's data is considered for the unit time step. In *Fig.* 3.1, the exponential curve fit to the actual data values is shown , along with their R^2 value. As seen in *Fig.* 3.1, the infection's growth rate is nonlinear (actual data points). Furthermore, mapping data points with a logistic regression curve suggests that the growth rate follows an exponential trend. The fact that the coefficient of determination (R^2) is close to 1 supports the logic, meaning that the fit closely aligns well with the actual data points. Equation 3.1, an exponential growth model equation, is used to determine the fit. The logistic parameters' values determine how close the modelled data curve is as compared to the real data curve. The chosen logistic parameter values are implicitly determined, and the best logistic fit for the actual dataset is represented.

The Logistic trajectory given by *Eq.* 3.2 appears to closely match the increasing pattern of growing Covid-19 cases. In all four regions, the R^2 estimator value (Coefficient of Determination) is near to one, indicating that the computed values based

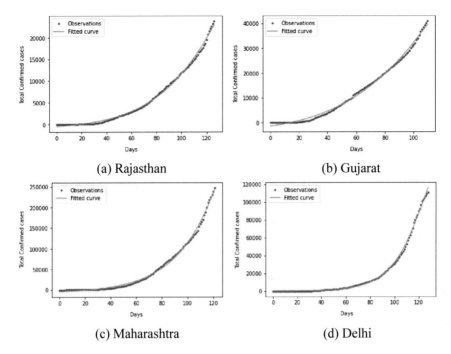

Fig. 3.1 Coefficient of determination (R^2) values-based comparison of actual and logistic curve for Rajasthan, Gujarat, Maharashtra, and Delhi. The R^2 values for these four location are 99.71%, 99.75%, 99.76%, and 99.81%, respectively

on the logistic relation are consistent with the genuine values. In each case, there is a slight variability in terms of growth rate and duration. However, each growth pattern follows a nearly identical upward trajectory, implying that the infection pattern can be predicted using real-valued data. As a result, the same concept can be used in a variety of diverse circumstances.

Similar to the infection growth trend, the trend of recovery rate also follows the exponential trajectory. Figure 3.2 represents the recovery trend graphs for the four regions (Rajasthan, Gujarat, Maharashtra, and Delhi) of India based on the data taken from [2]. The curvature for all the graphs defines an exponential increment of the recovery rate from the disease. This is very much analogous to the infection growth trend. For this analysis, the data has been considered for the period from mid of *February* 2020 to *August* 2020 end. The smoothness of the growing curves is not the same for all the four cases. Like for Delhi, the growth of the recovery graph shoots more aggressively just as the curve starts rising. This again can be seen as an effect of the growth in the infection trend. The infection growth trend curve of Delhi too has such sharp bending once the cases are on a rise. From this, we can relate the two processes of people getting infected and getting recovered in a manner that initially both the processes will start growing at a different rate following the exponential

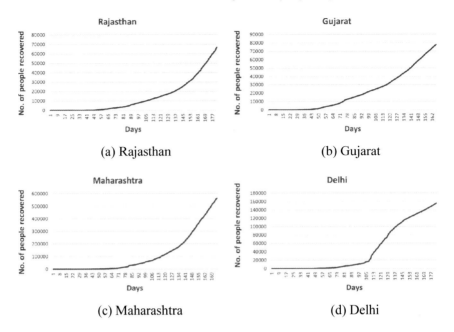

Fig. 3.2 Recovery growth rate trends for Rajasthan, Gujarat, Maharashtra, and Delhi, respectively

trajectory. After that, the infection curve tends to grow faster than the recovery trend and this continues till the entire or close to the entire population does not get infected. After this stage, the infection growth trend starts dipping and the recovery rate graph starts climbing up.

In analogy to the infection and recovery growth rate curves, the death rate curve too follows an exponential trajectory. Figure 3.3 shows the death rate tolls for the four states for the same period as of recovery rate. The smoothness of the trends is again not similar but the overall trajectory of the growth shows a multiplicative increase in the number of deaths. Interestingly, even the cusps and breaks in the curve too are very much similar in all the three cases for respective regions. This is enough to understand that the dynamics of the viral infection is exponential in nature and all its related event too follows an exponential trend. This allows us to think of the mathematical model in terms of an *exponential differential* model like the SIR (Susceptible, Infected, and Recovery) model which can capture and explain the dynamics of the disease well. But before proceeding towards the exploration of Covid-19 using the SIR model, let's discuss why *logistic regression*-based analysis of the disease is not adequate for drawing conclusions.

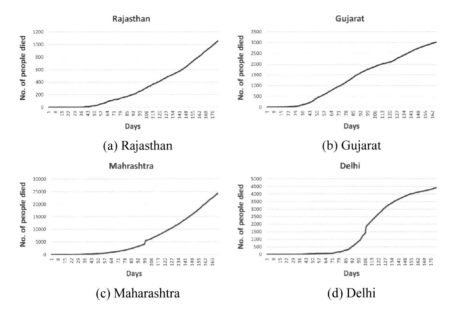

Fig. 3.3 Death growth rate trends for Rajasthan, Gujarat, Maharashtra, and Delhi, respectively

3.2 Need of SIR Model-Based Analysis for Covid-19

Although the model used to make the forecast appears to be adequate, it cannot be generalized because

1. The curvature of the disease graph tends to have an exponential advancement, but the smoothness of the curve, as shown, is not guaranteed. The sharp peaks in the cusp are caused by daily fluctuations in the number of people affected. Since different reasons (improved social distancing measures, good immunity, climate conditions, lower population density, and so on) are not considered by the model, some of the predictions may appear unrealistic.
2. Only the rate of infection over time is taken into account by the model. The underlying function takes a day number as an input and returns the predicted number of sick people for that day. Other considerations, such as recovery rate, the initial vulnerable persons, and so on, are all missing.
3. The trajectory is exponential because the initial growth trend of any viral infection like Covid-19 follows a multiplicative factor increment. However, in practice, no phenomenon exists that always has an upward inclination. When the number of cases remains stable given the rate of recovery is low, there will be a dip in the future. As a result, while the current model appears to be a decent predictive model, it is not analytically sound for making future predictions.

4. Other information, such as contamination rate, how long the infection persists after recovering patients, the influence of an increase in susceptibles at any point in time, and so on, cannot be obtained or anticipated using this simple growth model.

Thus, both recovered and vulnerable people's growth and their effects on each other need to be taken into account. As a result, we revisit the missing aspects in the following chapters of the book. The model presented in this chapter is adequate for determining the infection's general development tendency. So, in the rest of the chapters, an exponential differential model called the SIR model is presented to explain the missing aspects. It is due to the fact that modelling through SIR takes into consideration the susceptible counts, infected patients and recovered patients. The model equations try to draw out the relation in between these three model variables which was missing in the case of logistic regression analysis. In the case of logistic regression-based analysis, the trend analysis is accomplished individually for all the three aspects. And, hence, the effect of one variable or stage over another cannot be observed. More importantly, it just mimics the growth trend. For the current data trends, the fit looks good. But once the trajectory starts to dip, the same equation will not fit well to capture the sudden change in the dynamics of the curve.

References

1. COVID-19 Corona Virus India Dataset, Homepage: https://www.kaggle.com/imdevskp/covid19-corona-virus-india-dataset?select=complete.csv *by Devakumar Kp*, Accessed on 24/03/2022
2. Covid-19 in India, Homepage: https://www.kaggle.com/datasets/sudalairajkumar/covid19-in-india?select=covid_vaccine_statewise.csv, Accessed on 24/03/2022
3. Flutrackers.com Homepage: https://www.kaggle.com/imdevskp/covid19-corona-virus-india-dataset?select=complete.csv by Devakumar Kp, My red bolding, Accessed on 24/03/2022

Chapter 4
SIR Model-Based Experimental Investigations over Covid-19

In this chapter, simulations of real data have been conducted using the SIR model. The chapter also investigates the effect of lockdown for the four prominently Covid-19 hit areas of India. Afterwards, the estimated fraction of the population that will get infected is determined. The chapter contains visualizations showing how changing the model's parameters simulates curve growth.

4.1 Understanding SIR as a Nonlinear Differential Model

The SIR model [7], which considers a larger number of components and variables, is one of the most suitable disease modelling techniques. The SIR epidemic model is the foundation for all other epidemic models (SEIR and SIS). The Susceptible, Exposed, Infected, and Recovered (SEIR) model is an extension of the SIR model, with the exception that the *exposed population* is separated from the susceptibles at a later stage. However, for Covid-19, because of the very high infection spread rate, all the susceptibles can be considered as potentially exposed. As a result, susceptibles (S) in the population can be equated to the exposed phase (E). The third phase in the SIS model is *susceptible*, which indicates that after becoming infected, a person advances to the susceptible stage. But, given the disease's current trend, the chances of a patient becoming infected after a recovery are very low. People who once suffered from the disease will no longer be in the Susceptible (S) stage, according to the SIR model and the model has a separate Recovery (R) stage for recovered patients. Hence, in comparison to SIR, modelling the disease using the SIS model makes less sense.

As previously stated, SIR model-based evaluations are based on three factors: susceptible population, infected population, and recovered individuals. The rate of change of expressions of a number of susceptibles, infected, and recovered patients are as follows, as defined in Chap. 3:

R. Saxena et al., *Exploring Susceptible-Infectious-Recovered (SIR) Model for COVID-19 Investigation*, SpringerBriefs in Computational Intelligence, https://doi.org/10.1007/978-981-19-4175-7_4

$$\frac{dS}{dt} = -aSI \qquad (4.1)$$

$$\frac{dI}{dt} = aSI - bI \qquad (4.2)$$

$$\frac{dR}{dt} = bI \qquad (4.3)$$

Next, the model parameters are matched using these simple nonlinear differential equations. But first, let's go over a couple of terms:

- *Effective Contact rate (a):* It is calculated by multiplying the transmission rate by the contact rate. For example, if the transmission rate is 6% and 6 contacts are made per day, then the effective contact rate is $= 0.06 * 6 = 0.36$.
- *Recovery rate (b):* It is defined as the recovery period (average number of days) taken by a patient to recover from an infection. For example, if a patient's typical recovery time is 4 days, then the recovery rate is $= 1/4 = 0.25$.
- *Reproduction Number (R_0)* : Another term worth mentioning is R_0, which stands for reproduction number, defined by the ratio of a to b. The value intuitively conveys how quickly the epidemic spreads. The epidemic will not spread if the value of R_0 is 1. If the value is greater than one, the epidemic is likely to spread. The epidemic spread rate grows more aggressive as the value of R_0 above this rises.

At time 't,' *Eq.* 4.2 gives the number of vulnerable people who are infected minus the number of affected people who recovered from the virus. The effective contact rate of the conversion of susceptible to infected is represented by a, while the recovery rate is represented by b. The initial rate of change can be calculated using *Eq.* 4.3

$$\frac{dI}{dt_{t=0}} = aS_0 b - bI_0 \qquad (4.4)$$

The reproduction rate, given as R_0, is specified by the factor $\frac{aS_0}{b}$. Here, S_0 represents the initial susceptible population, a defines the transmission rate, and the recovery rate is denoted by b. In this mathematical expression, R_0 is a measure of the disease's contagiousness. It indicates the average number of people that an infected person can infect before recovery. Consider effective contact rate ($a = 0.06$) (transmission rate being 1% and 6 contacts are made per day) and recovery rate ($b = \frac{1}{15}$). Now, $R_0 = 0.06 \times 15 = 0.9$, i.e. on an average 10 infected people can infect 9 others, or 100 people can infect 90 others.

There are three possibilities based on the value of R_0:

- If $R_0 < 1$, the infectious individual will infect less than a person. This implies that the virus's spread starts dying and eventually cease.

- If $R_0 = 1$, the infectious person will infect only one individual in this situation. Here, the disease will continue to exist, but will not take the form epidemic.
- In this situation, if $R_0 > 1$, the infected person will infect more than one people, resulting in an epidemic/pandemic.

The magnitude of R_0 value fluctuates based on severity of a disease's viral infection. Influenza epidemic of 1918 flu (Spanish flu) was predicted to have a R_0 value of 1.4–2.8 [3]. Similarly, Swine flu and H1N1 flu have R_0 value in the range of 1.4–1.6. In *Sect.* 5.3, a more extensive comparison view is presented. According to the study reported in [9], the R_0 value considered for Covid-19 is in the range of 5.7–6.3 (based on the data of the first outbreak in Wuhan, China). The value of R_0 was formerly given 1.8–3.0; however, this range was later eliminated in [9].

The model's analytical results are based on the disease's R_0 value. It is ultimately determined by the number of contacts made and their frequency. The R_0 value for Covid-19 (5.7–6.3), as reported by [9], takes into account a variety of biological, socio-behavioural as well as environmental factors that influence virus transmission. However, because there is no direct metric for estimating the value of R_0, it is given based on mathematical observations. The influence of the R_0 value, rather than how the R_0 value is calculated, makes more sense in the context of the reported simulations and analytical results.

As $R_0 = \frac{aS_0}{b}$, the dependent parameters on which the value of R_0 depends are transmission rate (a) and recovery rate (b), where S_0 is a constant that represents the initial susceptible population. For different diseases, the 'a' and 'b' factors have varying values. Theoretically, $a > 0$ and $b > 0$ hold true because both the parameters are bound to have non-negative values. When $a >> b$, the value of R_0 is high, which explains the high rate of viral spread. If $b >> a$, it indicates that the epidemic is nearing its end. In practice, analysing the value of a and b parameters is difficult because these variables differ region-wise as well as country-wise. Furthermore, as per [6], they are dependent on several uncontrolled aspects such as people's social distancing measures, regional immunity, temperature and weather conditions, and so on. However, given the transmission rate (a) and R_0 value, b is estimated to be about 1/15 based on the analysis in [10] and [8]. This suggests that if each individual is infected for 15 days, we can anticipate 1/15th of those infected to recover each day. The R_0 value varies from 1.1 to 3.8, with 0.073–0.2533 as the effective contact rate. On the contrary, in several other countries and regions, the effective contact rate ranges from 0.38 to 0.42, resulting in a R_0 value of 5.7–6.3.

The number for recovery rate is chosen as *1/15* for the sake of feasibility, and R_0 is assumed to be 6.0 as per [9]. The value of R_0 can change (can go up or down). The value is determined by the variation in infection and recovery rates. To illustrate this, the graph in *Fig.* 4.1 depicts how a generic SIR model will expand.

The following values are found in the growth model: recovery rate = 1/15 and effective contact rate 0.4. The value of $R_0 = 6.0$ is derived from this. Experimental simulations have been carried out over a population of 1000 people using these values for equation parameters. The disease spreads quickly at first because of the high R_0 value, but as time passes, the number of people who are susceptible decreases.

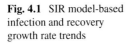

Fig. 4.1 SIR model-based infection and recovery growth rate trends

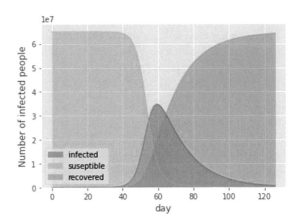

Furthermore, when more infected individuals finish their recovery time, the growth rate of infection decreases. As a result, the graph of the recovery phase heads up. This declines the rate of infection in people, but it is still strong enough. This trend declines exponentially with time after attaining the peak.

4.2   Analysing Lockdown Effect on Effective Contact Rate: An Experimental Simulation over Covid-19 Data

The trend for the Rajasthan state's curve is shown in *Fig.* 4.2. It is derived using the same parameter values. The experimental simulations have been conducted over a period of 78 days, and the day of the first Corona-positive patient was discovered until the 20th of May, 2020. Three factors of Covid-19 development are considered:

- *Infected*: The red line curve in every graph from *Figs.* 4.2, 4.3, 4.4, and 4.5 reflects the count of infected patients predicted by applying the SIR model for the given R_0 value ($= 6.0$).
- *Actual Data Trend*: The purple line in *Figs.* 4.2, 4.3, 4.4, and 4.5 indicates the trend in the number of people becoming infected by Covid-19.
- $Infected_{lockdown}$: This reflects the deviation of the growth trend of contagion from the model prognosis for the real data. This helps in determining the crucial role that lockdown has played in order to lower the contact rate, as depicted by the blue line curve in Figs. 4.2 and 4.5.

The red curve reflects that by the 25th day of the start of infection, the infected people count shoots above 10000, according to the SIR model growth equations, starting with an initial population 80 million people approximately as per [5]. The *purple* growing line, on the other hand, depicts the real growth rate of infected

Fig. 4.2 Lockdown analysis curve for Rajasthan

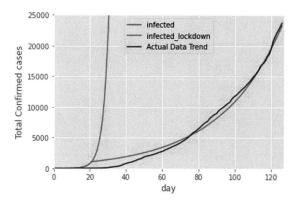

Fig. 4.3 Lockdown analysis curve for Maharashtra

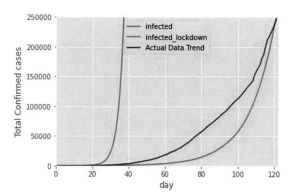

patients. As a result, it can be deduced that something was done in the meantime to reduce the number of contacts by the infected people.

Now, consider increase in S_0 by a factor of 'S' where $S > 0$. Then $\frac{(aS_0+S)}{b} > \frac{aS_0}{b}$. As a result, the contagion growth increases with the rise in susceptibles count. This scenario has arisen as a result of the fact that some migrants who were not included in the first population census have returned to their hometowns during this period.

Here, the data in consideration is from 24th of March, 2020, when India was under a shutdown state, which lasted till the 20th of May, 2020. The blue curve line (refer to Fig. 4.2) depicts a shift in the trajectory. The blue line follows the original model trajectory until the 21st day, after which the *effective contact rate* was reduced by a factor of 4.175. As a result, the lockdown was successful in suppressing the growth trend until the 78th day. After 78th day, this reduction was a little closer to 4.19, but later on due to the increased growth rate of Covid-19 in the state, the overall reduction effect can be considered to be around 4.175. A similar analysis is carried out on the Maharashtra and Gujarat datasets, which may be found in *Figs.* 4.3 and 4.4, respectively.

The number of susceptibles in Maharashtra is identified as 124.9 million people, which is the total population according to census [4]. As compared to the curve

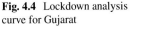

Fig. 4.4 Lockdown analysis curve for Gujarat

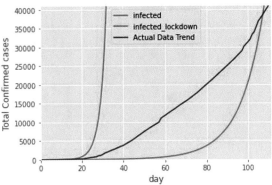

of Fig. 4.2, the real Covid-19 data growth rate is fairly high here, depicted by the *purple* line curvature. Initially, the growth rate of the curvature is relatively slow, and about the 30th day, the curvature starts to shoot up. According to the SIR model, the predicted growth rate is having extremely rapid growth, as seen by the *red* line. Lockdown was implemented after 15 days since the very first positive patient was detected in Maharashtra. So, the overall effective contact rate reduced 2.45 times which can be observed by the growth of the blue line.

With a similar explanation, the effective contact rate was cut down to 1.955 after the lockdown for Gujarat state for a population of 65 million according to the census for Gujarat [2]. It is not as much as it has been for Rajasthan and Maharashtra. As a result, the total number of cases reported (in Gujarat) had risen to more than 11, 500 as on the 62nd day. Throughout the graph, the growth rate shown by the purple line (denoting the actual data) is found to be higher than the blue line (denoting the modified model curve). This suggests an effective contact rate reduction by a factor of 1.955 times, indicating the lateral impacts of lockdown in Gujarat.

Delhi's effective contact shrinks by a factor of about 4.5 for the specified R_0 value 6.0 and for 30.2 million people [1]. As can be seen in *Fig.* 4.1, the preliminary outbreak in Delhi was powerful, but due to lockdown, it was unable to grow at a pace shown by the red line. But still, the rate of disease transmission remained significant.

Irregular gaping between the blue line and the purple line in different states is influenced by a variety of factors. In comparison to other locations, the infection spread began substantially early in certain regions. As a result, the infection rates prior and post lockdown differ significantly for these regions. Another aspect is that the lockdown's influence over the contact rate is not uniform across all the regions. This characteristic is uncontrollable because it is dependent on the inhabitants of the underlying region's social distancing strategies. This can be observed in Maharashtra and Gujarat where the propagation of infection was aggressive for the initial contagion. This can be observed as the bigger gap between the blue and the purple line in the last two curves (Figs. 4.4 and 4.5).

Fig. 4.5 Lockdown analysis
curve for Delhi

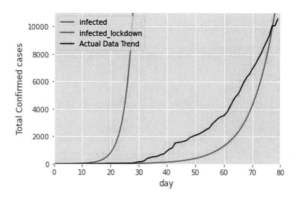

4.3 Summarizing Analysis

The following is a list of findings based on the foregoing discussion:

- The SIR model is defined as a nonlinear differential equation model explained by
  Eq. 4.4, which is an exponential growth model. Because of the continual reduction
  in the R_0 factor due to lockdown, the growth trends in Figs. 4.2, 4.3, 4.4, and 4.5, the
  blue and purple line converge towards each other. This accounts for nonlinearity
  in the curvature.
- The model dynamics do not completely match the growth trend. This is owing to
  a changing infection growth rate caused by the population's susceptibility dimin-
  ishing at an unpredictable rate. This is because a lot of people travelled to their
  hometowns during the lockdown period. It is assumed that the susceptible population would remain constant. The rate of infection is directly related to this
  parameter. To demonstrate this mathematically, as per Eq. 4.4, in which the condition in which an epidemic will continue to spread is represented by

$$\frac{a S_0}{b} > 1$$

For this, consider that S_0 is incremented by an additional 's' population where
$s > 0$, then

$$\frac{a(S_0 + s)}{b} > \frac{a S_0}{b}$$

This means that as the susceptible count increases, so does the number of infected
people. As shown by Eq. 4.4, the rise will be exponential. This scenario has arisen as
a result of the fact that some migrants who were not included in the first population
census have returned to their hometowns during this period.

- Furthermore, the aforementioned cases lead us to the conclusion that the tuning
  parameters are the key to guide the model's prediction abilities. The *effective
  contact rate, a*; *recovery rate, b*; and the *number of Susceptibles, S* serve as the

tuning parameters. Corresponding to these parameters, a few critical properties are listed as follows:

- 'S' is kept constant since the population during the first lockdown has not been vaccinated against the viral outbreak, the entire population was at risk of being infected. As a result of the above argument, the epidemic depends on two components, a and b, and the R_0 equation for epidemic growth is updated to

$$\frac{a}{b} > 1$$

  Since the rate of recovery is nearly constant, fifteen days, the only variable left to consider is the *effective contact rate*. As the effective contact rate decreases, the equation inequality tends towards a value lower than 1, as the effective contact rate decreases. Because of this, the implementation of lockdown in all the states helped them to limit the outbreak (since the outbreak did not spread at the rate predicted by the SIR model with R_0 value = 6.0).
- As the rate of contagion begins to flatten or decline, the recovery rate begins to rise. This is because more and more number of infected people are recovered now as compared to newly infected people.
- The transmission of the virus is not affected by the total population value. It is determined by the initial infected population and the disease's R_0 value. Considering Delhi's infection growth rate curve, this notion can be understood well. In contrast to other states, the infection rate in Delhi was substantially higher (see Fig. 4.5). Given that Delhi's population is small in contrast to other states, the actual infection count closely matched the SIR model estimations for the first few days. As a result, even if the population is dense, the epidemic outbreak will be mild due to the disease's low R_0 value and the less number of people suffering from the disease, initially.

Till now, the discussion has focused on how well the SIR model simulates the actual growth data and what conclusions may be taken from deviations from the trend. The further in-depth analysis of SIR modelling over the four states is discussed in the next chapter.

References

1. Delhi Population, Homepage: http://www.populationu.com/in/delhi-population, Accessed on 24/03/2022
2. Gujarat Population, Homepage: http://www.populationu.com/in/gujarat-population, Accessed on 24/03/2022
3. Healthline, Homepage: https://www.healthline.com/health/r-naught-reproduction-number, Accessed on 24/03/2022
4. Maharashtra Population, Homepage: https://www.census2011.co.in/census/state/maharashtra.html, Accessed on 24/03/2022

5. Rajasthan Population, Homepage: http://www.populationu.com/in/rajasthan-population, Accessed on 24/03/2022
6. Delamater, P.L., Street, E.J., Leslie, T.F., Tony Yang, Y., Jacobsen, K.H.: Complexity of the basic reproduction number (r0). Emerg. Infect. Dis. **25**(1,) 1 (2019)
7. Dworkin, J., Tan, S.Y.: Ronald ross (1857–1932): discoverer of malaria's life cycle. Singapore Med. J. **52**(7), 466–467 (2011)
8. Patil, K., Murali, A., Ganguli, P., Nandi, S., Sarkar, R.R.: Temporal analysis of covid-19 pandemic in India and r0 prediction (2020)
9. Sanche, S., Ting Lin, Y., Xu, C., Romero-Severson, E., Hengartner, N., Ke., R.: High contagiousness and rapid spread of severe acute respiratory syndrome coronavirus 2. Emerg. Infect. Dis., **26**(7), 1470–1477 (2020)
10. Shinde, G.R., Kalamkar, A.B., Mahalle, P.N., Dey, N., Chaki, J., Hassanien, A.E.: Forecasting models for coronavirus disease (covid-19): a survey of the state-of-the-art. SN Comput. Sci. **1**(4), 1–15 (2020)

Chapter 5
Result Analysis of SIR-Based Covid-19 Model

After collecting insights from *Chap.* 4, several facets of Covid-19 modelling have been explored in this chapter. For the four Indian regions chosen, a maximum number of infected people are predicted. Parameters connected to the pandemic's end are also estimated. Estimations associated with the vaccination process and herd immunity have been proposed. The estimated computations are based on the SIR-defined nonlinear differential equation model. Fundamental calculus ideas and simple curve analysis have been used to generate these estimations from the well-defined SIR differential equation model.

5.1 SIR Model-Based Estimation of Infection Range

Considering Eqs. 4.1 and 4.2 from *Chap.* 4, we have

$$\frac{dS}{dt} = -aSI \text{ and } \frac{dI}{dt} = aSI - bI$$

Dividing these two equations, we have

$$\frac{dI}{dS} = -\frac{aSI - bI}{aSI}$$

$$\frac{dI}{dS} = -1 + \frac{1}{R_0 . S}$$

where $R_0 = a/b$. Solving it further using integral calculus, the infected number of persons at any time 't' can be given as

$$I + S - \frac{1}{R_0} \ln S = I_0 + S_0 - \frac{1}{R_0} \ln S_0 \tag{5.1}$$

© The Author(s), under exclusive license to Springer Nature Singapore Pte Ltd. 2022
R. Saxena et al., *Exploring Susceptible-Infectious-Recovered (SIR) Model for COVID-19 Investigation*, SpringerBriefs in Computational Intelligence,
https://doi.org/10.1007/978-981-19-4175-7_5

Here, S_0 is the initial susceptible population and I_0 is the initial infected population at time t = 0. Maximum value of Eq. 5.1 occurs at a point where $\frac{dI}{dt} = 0$ as it is a monotonically increasing curve. Thus, calculating derivative of Eq. 5.1 with respect to 't', we have

$$S = \frac{b}{a} = \frac{1}{R_0} \tag{5.2}$$

Putting this value in Eq. 5.1 and rearranging terms, the maximum infected population by the disease can be estimated as

$$I_{max} = I_0 + S_0 - \frac{1}{R_0}(1 + \ln R_0.S_0) \tag{5.3}$$

Equation 5.3 expresses the greatest number of people who will become infected as a result of the virus's propagation. The entire equation can be expressed using only a single variable, R_0. Hence, for the sake of feasibility, it is assumed that the value of R_0 remained constant throughout this analysis. Given that the implementation of lockdown has reduced R_0, the maximum fraction of the population infected is shown in Table 5.1, assuming b, i.e. the recovery rate to be constant and initially the entire population is susceptible.

The actual statistics may differ slightly from the expected numbers. This is because of model assumptions like the following: (i) The model considers the susceptible count equal to the entire population count. (ii) The model assumes constant values of effective contact rate and recovery rate. If any of these factors change in the middle, estimated values of I_{max} will also change. Stronger social distancing mechanisms would limit the effective contact rate as a result of increasing awareness; therefore, this is extremely likely to happen over a period of time. As a result, the number of people who can become infected will be reduced. The number of susceptible people will be lowered significantly if the underlying population is vaccinated aggressively.

Table 5.1 Predicting I_{max}

State	Population	R_0 value before lockdown	I_{max} estimate based on original R_0 value	R_0 value after lockdown	I_{max} estimate based on new R_0 value
Rajasthan	80 million [4]	6.0	78.80 million	6.0/4.175 = 1.437	76 million
Gujarat	65 million [2]	6.0	63.838 million	6.0/1.98 = 3.030	62.926 million
Maharashtra	124 million [3]	6.0	122.73 million	6.0/2.45 = 2.44	122.49 million
Delhi	30.2 million [1]	6.0	29.166 million	6.0/4.5 = 1.333	26.67 million

Another missing aspect is the availability and invention of drugs to cure the Covid-19 can improve the recovery rate significantly. As a result, the model's outcome offers a sense of Covid-19 trend's aggressiveness, not the exact precise estimations. Furthermore, given the present infection trend, it also reveals which regions require quick care. It is clear from the table that despite its small population Gujarat needs more immediate care than Rajasthan.

5.2 To Estimate Longevity of Covid-19 Pandemic Spread

With the progress in the pandemic spread, the total number of people who are susceptible begins to decline in proportion to the entire population. The monotonically growing curve of the infected population reaches its peak value which is corresponding to the condition $S = b/a$, as determined by Eq. 5.1.

The infected population curve begins to drop after this point, and the trajectory follows the curve depicted in *Fig.* 5.1 as per the SIR model. As a result, after a significant amount of time (time tends to infinity), for $b >> a$, implying that S is approximately equal to b. The statement means that practically everyone who was infected has recovered. The number of infected people is quite low at this stage, and the expression for $R_0 = a/b$ indicates that the pandemic is nearing its end.

One can deduce from this discussion that the end of an epidemic is determined by the absence of infected individuals rather than the absence of susceptibles in the population. To put it another way, the recovery rate is much larger than the infection rate as the pandemic nears its end. This is yet another reality that can be mathematically illuminated as well as can be deduced from data.

Fig. 5.1 SIR Growth Model

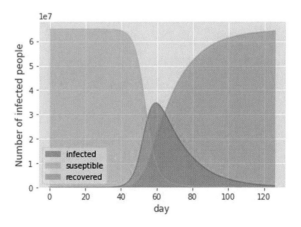

5.3   Comparing Covid-19 with Other Epidemics

Covid-19's growth is compared to several other epidemics. As per the literature, the Covid-19 is highly contagious [9, 10] (with reproduction number almost equal to 6.0). The R_0 values for different diseases are shown in Table 5.2, as per [5].

Figure 5.2 is the result of an experiment conducted on a 5, 000 population sample. For each infection, the upper limit of the R_0 value is considered, e.g. 18 for Measles, 1.08 for SARS, and so on. The rehabilitation period for all diseases is considered to be 15 days for the purpose of simplicity. Figure 5.3 depicts the growth of several diseases using these parameter values and the SIR Model. In the case of measles, the disease spreads very rapidly due to its high R_0 value and around 90% of the people get infected. The growth tendency and range of all other diseases are not as aggressive as measles. However, the Covid-19 rise is considerable owing to the high R_0 value, especially in densely populated regions.

Comparing the Covid-19 pandemic to the epidemics and pandemics like influenza, the most significant difference is that the other pandemics have systems in place to decrease the number of people who are susceptible. As a result, peak achievement for diseases like measles will differ from what is portrayed in the image, and the

Table 5.2   Diseases and their R_0 values

Disease name	R_0 value
SARS	0.19–1.08
Measles	12–18
Ebola	1.5–1.9
Influenza (1918 Pandemic)	1.4–2.8
Nipah [8]	0.1–0.4
MERS	0.3-0.8

Fig. 5.2   Graphical Plot of I_{max} estimation for different diseases

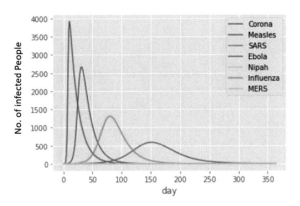

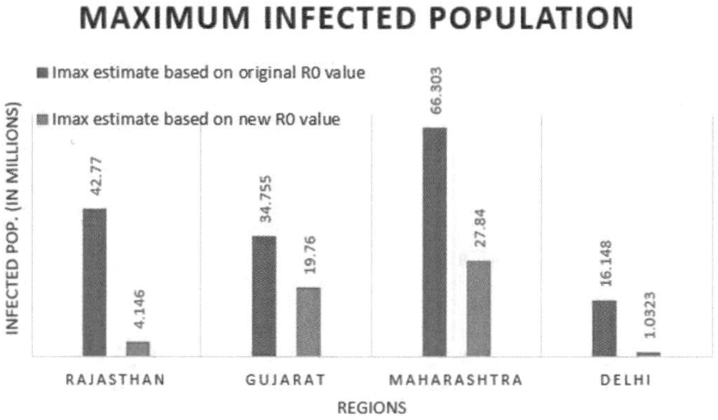

MAXIMUM INFECTED POPULATION

Fig. 5.3 SIR Model-based simulation to evaluate maximum infected people for different diseases

vaccine may be used to effectively combat the underlying disease. According to data from [6], herd immunity and immunization will prevent the disease from spreading like wildfire.

Containment is attainable, and the disease will soon be eradicated thanks to these handling mechanisms and safety precautions. Though the death rate of Covid-19 is not as high as that of Ebola [11] and Nipah [7], these diseases are less lethal than Covid-19 because they do not have such a high degree of contamination. Covid-19 is still a long way from achieving herd immunity due to a lack of known treatment options. As a result, the overall impact of Covid-19 is still worse than diseases like Nipah and Ebola. Regardless of how high the death rate and contamination are, the significance of vaccination and herd immunity is highly relevant to this context. By vaccinating a segment of the population, the disease's spread can be limited and a portion of the population can be saved from the disease. Furthermore, as time passes, herd immunity (development of anti-bodies against the disease) becomes more important.

5.4   Covid-19 Curbing Measures: Vaccination v/s Herd Immunity

Even if it is assumed that the vaccine is 100 percent effective, it is prohibitively expensive to vaccinate all the people. Furthermore, some people may have a weakened immune system and will be unable to get vaccinated. Is there a way to assure that the pandemic spread is controlled by vaccinating a population fraction? And the answer is yes. It can be simply deduced from an analysis of the SIR model. Herd immunity is the answer to the question. Let 'p' be the proportion of the population who is vaccinated. The people who are vaccinated will be $p \times S_0$. This quantity will be removed from S_0 assuming 100% effectiveness of the vaccine. The remaining

Table 5.3 Prediction of population to be vaccinated

State	Population	Current R_0 value after lockdown	Population to be vaccinated $((1 - \frac{1}{R_0}) *$ Population)
Rajasthan	80 million [4]	1.437	24.32 million
Gujarat	65 million [2]	3.030	43.54 million
Maharashtra	124 million [3]	2.44	73.180 million
Delhi	30.2 million [1]	1.333	7.544 million

susceptibles will now be determined as $(1 - p).S_0$, and hence, the relationship between a, b, p, and S_0 can be defined as

$$(1 - p).S_0 \frac{a}{b} \leq 1$$

After further simplification,

$$(1 - p)\frac{a}{b} \leq \frac{1}{S_0}$$

$R_0 = \frac{a S_0}{b}$ (from Chap. 4). Thus, at equilibrium, we have

$$(1 - p) = \frac{1}{R_0}$$

and, finally, we have,

$$p = 1 - \frac{1}{R_0} \tag{5.4}$$

Finally, Eq. 5.4 gives the fraction of the population that needs to be vaccinated (p). The value of R_0 has a direct impact on the solution p. The related p value(s) will change in response to changes in the R_0 value(s). Estimations for the states are shown in Table 5.3, based on the existing R_0 values that sustain the rate of infection growth as mentioned above in Table 5.1.

Another thing to consider is vaccine efficacy. If the R_0 value is 2.0 and the entire vulnerable population is 1000, the fraction of the population that has to be vaccinated is $1000/2.0 = 500$. However, if the vaccine is considered 90% effective, then this number will be $500/0.9 = 556$. As a result, the vaccine's efficacy has an impact on herd immunity and vaccination.

References

1. Delhi Population, Homepage: http://www.populationu.com/in/delhi-population, Accessed on 24/03/2022
2. Gujarat Population, Homepage: http://www.populationu.com/in/gujarat-population, Accessed on 24/03/2022

3. Maharashtra Population, Homepage: https://www.census2011.co.in/census/state/maharashtra.html, Accessed on 24/03/2022
4. Rajasthan Population, Homepage: http://www.populationu.com/in/rajasthan-population, Accessed on 24/03/2022
5. Delamater, P.L., Street, E.J., Leslie, T.F., Tony Yang, Y., Jacobsen, K.H.: Complexity of the basic reproduction number (r0). Emerg. Infect. Dis. **25**(1), 1 (2019)
6. Huremović, D.: Brief history of pandemics (pandemics throughout history). In: Psychiatry of Pandemics, pp. 7–35. Springer (2019)
7. Longdon, B., Hadfield, J.D., Day, J.P., Smith, S.C.L., McGonigle, J.E., Cogni, R., Cao, C., Jiggins, F.M.: The causes and consequences of changes in virulence following pathogen host shifts. PLoS Pathog **11**(3), e1004728 (2015)
8. Mondal, M.K., Hanif, M., Ali Biswas, M.H.: A mathematical analysis for controlling the spread of nipah virus infection. Int. J. Modell. Simul. **37**(3), 185–197 (2017)
9. Nesteruk, I.: Estimations of the coronavirus epidemic dynamics in South Korea with the use of sir model. Preprint.] ResearchGate (2020)
10. Russo, L., Anastassopoulou, C., Tsakris, A., Bifulco, G.N., Campana, E.F., Toraldo, G., Siettos, C.: Tracing DAY-ZERO. forecasting the fade out of the covid-19 outbreak in lombardy. Italy: a compartmental modelling and numerical optimization approach (2020)
11. Shah, S., Das, S., Jain, A., Misra, D.P., Negi, V.S.: A systematic review of the prophylactic role of chloroquine and hydroxychloroquine in coronavirus disease-19 (covid-19). Int. J. Rheum. Dis. **235**, 613–619 (2020)

Chapter 6
Exploring Covid-19 Second Wave Dynamics Using SIR Epidemic Model

This chapter illustrates the SIR model-based exploration of the second wave dynamics of Covid-19 for the same selected regions of India. The chapter explains the model-based variability in the growth trend, lockdown impact, vaccination, herd immunity, etc. drawing parallels with the first wave dynamics of Covid-19. Based on these lines, the chapter presents the following aspects:

- Covid-19 second wave: Emergence and Growth.
- Impact of lockdown 2.0.
- Comparing the two waves of Covid-19.
- Vaccination measures and its effect.

6.1 Covid-19 Second Wave: Impact, Emergence, and Growth

The infection rate preceding the first wave effect of Covid-19 was a steady, gradual decline. Post-March in 2021 [12], the infection again started to climb up gradually and was on a high in the April first week. The variant is termed as Covid-19 *Delta Variant*. The variant was found to be highly aggressive in comparison to the initial Covid-19 infection in 2019−20. Till 11th March, 2022, the Delta Variant had spread quickly across 170 countries [14]. The variant was aggressive enough to immediately call for action of *lockdown* in various countries. As per [13], the contagion of this new variant of Covid-19, named *B*.1.617.2 by the clinical experts, is 60% more than the previous viral infection. In India, the first case of this variant was found in December 2020 [14]. According to the American Society for Microbiology (ASM) [10], this new Delta stain was responsible for 83% of cases in the United States and 90% in the United Kingdom during the second wave. Also, as per ASM, as compared to the alpha variant, the delta variant's transmissibility is 40–60% more. At the same time, the alpha variant itself was 200% more contagious as compared to the original Wuhan

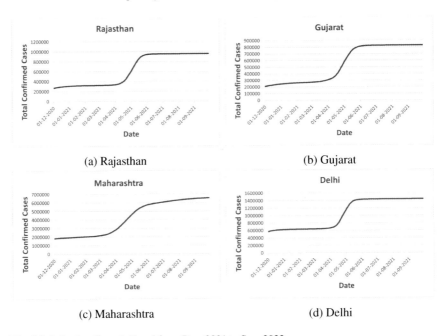

(a) Rajasthan   (b) Gujarat

(c) Maharashtra   (d) Delhi

Fig. 6.1 Infection Growth Trend from Dec. 2021 to Sep. 2022

stain [10]. Both contagion as well as fatality rates increased substantially faster, even though the second wave occurred over a much shorter period. According to WHO [8], the first wave registered $5, 001, 049$ cases whereas $5, 703, 208$ cases were reported during the second wave. The first wave's peak death count was $101, 084$, compared to $96, 684$ in the second wave. The first wave gradually started in March until it swiftly jumped (rapid infections) from October 2020 to February 2021, whereas the second wave rapidly surged from February 2021 to approximately June 2021. According to [4], the delta variant had a 108 per cent higher risk of hospitalization, a 235 per cent higher risk of ICU admission, and a 133 per cent higher risk of death than the original Wuhan variant.

Considering the regions of India (Rajasthan, Gujarat, Maharashtra, and Delhi), the contagion growth trends are as shown in Fig. 6.1 based on data from [2].

The growing trend of the infection is typically the same in all the regions and follows a general exponential rise. The growth trend of the disease was gradual till February 2021. After that, a sudden upsurge can be seen in the graph. The transition in the case of Delhi is quite sharp as compared to the other three regions. For Maharashtra, although the change is not abrupt enough, the exponential rise elongates even after the last data point, i.e. after 30th September, 2022. Further, all the curves appear to fit well to the logistic curve trajectory defined by the equation:

$$y = \frac{a}{1 + e^{-c(x-d)}} + b \qquad (6.1)$$

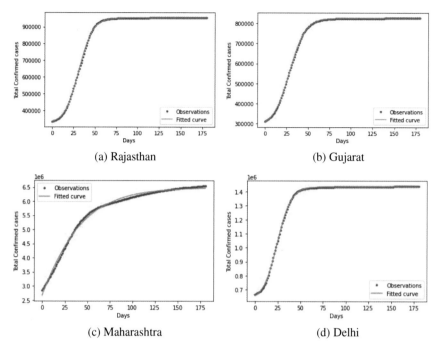

Fig. 6.2 Exponential Growth of Infection (April'21 to Sept.'21) with predicted R^2 values of 99.8%, 99.99%, 99.54%, and 99.97%, respectively

The alarming conditions appeared in India in the mid of March 2021 and from mid-April 2021 during which the lockdown was imposed in almost every state and region of the country. Carefully observing the growing curvatures of these four regions for the period from 1st March 2021 to 1st July 2021, it is realized that the actual data follows a logistic equation-based growth pattern. To analyse this, a simple logistic curve simulation has been carried out for the confirmed cases for each region. The data for the areas have been considered from 1st April 2021 to 29th September 2021, as this was the period in which the cases increased at a very rapid pace. This fast growth trend for Rajasthan, Gujarat, Maharashtra, and Delhi is shown in Fig. 6.2.

The growth trend of infection for all the four regions (Rajasthan, Gujarat, Maharashtra, and Delhi) suggests a perfect fit to the *logistic regression* curve with the predicted coefficient of determination (R^2) of 99.8%, 99.99%, 99.54%, and 99.97%, respectively. This is analogous to what has been discussed in Chap. 3 of the book, which implies that the growth pattern of any epidemic or pandemic grows exponentially.

Here, the curves differ in the shapes of their growth trajectory a bit. However, after attaining a peak, it is observed that the curve flattens. The exponential growth rate nearly becomes constant owing to certain factors like vaccination, strict lockdown protocols, development of herd immunity, etc. Only in the case of Maharashtra, does the curve continues to grow due to a large number of peoples in comparison to other states residing closely. Overall, the incline speed is highly acute and starts from the same point. However, the lockdown dates are different for different states this time since lockdowns were announced at the state levels (by the state governments, and hence, there is a variation). But still, the duration was almost the same, differing by a week or so.

For all the states, the initial infection rate was also exponential. This justifies that the initial growth trend of the pandemics or epidemics follows an exponential (logistic regression) growth trajectory. However, as discussed in Chap. 3, the exponential growth trend happens only in the initial phase. Still, for overall trend analysis of the pandemic, some more concrete mathematics is required as no process in the real world is completely exponential. Moreover, the logistic regression can only say about the growing trend. Other dynamics like how long the pandemic will stay, vaccination and herd immunity effect over infection, etc. cannot be explained or estimated based on logistic regression. The pandemic's behaviour majorly depends upon the contact rate and the contagion factor of the disease, which logistic regression does not consider.

6.2   Impact of Lockdown 2.0

In this section, SIR epidemic model dynamics have been investigated over the second wave of Covid-19. The *Reproduction Number*, (R_0) value of the *Delta* variant is reported to be almost two times as aggressive in comparison to the previous R_0 value, as per our discussion in the previous section. However, the measure of R_0 value differs from region to region and country to country. For the sake of our analysis, it has been considered that the delta stain is 60% more aggressive in comparison to the *alpha* variant [4]. Based on this, the R_0 value of the Delta variant is $R_0 = 6 + 0.6 * 6 = 9.6$. Considering the case of Rajasthan where a complete lockdown was imposed on 17th April, 2021 in order to counter the growing cases. Rajasthan was under a full lockdown state except for the necessary services to be operated, and officials associated with these services were allowed to move out. This lockdown was uplifted gradually after a duration of approximately 46 days. However, till 8th June, 2021, almost all the states of the country had lifted up the complete lockdown and had allowed controlled movement with Covid-19 protocols to be followed. Given this, Fig. 6.3 depicts the SIR model-based Covid-19 spread of the cases in Rajasthan. The experimental simulations have been conducted over a period of 128 days, from 1st February 2021 to 8th June, 2021. The reason for choosing this duration is that February marked the beginning of a severe eruption of cases which forced the governments to take a strong decision of another lockdown from mid of April. This continued till June and in June first week almost every state pulls off the decision. Three factors of Covid-19 development in the graph have been considered:

Fig. 6.3 Analysis curve for Rajasthan

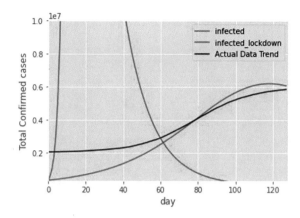

- *Infected*: The red line curves in the graphs from Figs. 6.3, 6.4, 6.5, and 6.6 reflect the number of infected patients anticipated by applying the Susceptible, Infectious, and/or Recovered (SIR) model for the given R_0 value (= 9.6).
- *Actual Data Trend*: This is depicted by the purple line in the graphical plots from Figs. 6.3, 6.4, 6.5, and 6.6, which indicates the pattern of the actual number of people becoming sick (due to Covid-19).
- *Infected_lockdown*: This graph depicts the evolution of the infection curvature as compared to the SIR model-based prognosis. The plots from Figs. 6.3, 6.4, 6.5, and 6.6 help to determine by the end of lockdown how much the effective contact rate has been reduced.

Consider the figure shown in Fig. 6.3 for Rajasthan state. The SIR with $R_0 = 9.6$ based red line curve indicates that given such a high R_0 value, the total population of the state may have been infected by 10th day from the start of infection. The *purple* growing line depicts the actual growth rate of infected patients. The difference in the

Fig. 6.4 Analysis curve for Maharashtra

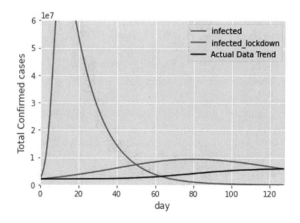

Fig. 6.5 Analysis curve for Gujarat

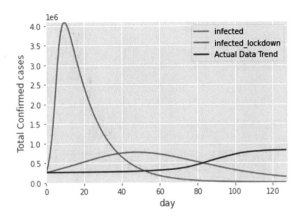

Fig. 6.6 Analysis curve for Delhi

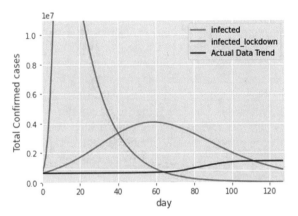

growth trajectory of the two lines suggests that some preventive measures had been taken to stop the growth rate of infection at a rate indicated by the red line.

The trajectory of the blue line (refer to Fig. 6.3) depicts a shift. The line touches the original trajectory represented in purple by the end of the lockdown, which suggests that the value of *effective contact rate* was reduced by a factor of *6.1*. As a result, the lockdown was successful in suppressing the growth trend from the 53rd day onwards from the start of the lockdown. A similar analysis is carried out on the Maharashtra, Gujarat, and Delhi datasets, which can be seen in Figs. 6.4, 6.5, and 6.6, respectively [2].

In the instance of Maharashtra, the growth rate is relatively high, as represented by the *purple line* of curvature. The SIR model shows this through the blue line curvature (SIR model-based growth prediction with reduced R_0 value). The initial growth rate of the curvature is relatively slow, and about on the 10th day, the curvature starts to shoot up. According to the model, real growth will be extraordinarily rapid (without lockdown), as evidenced by the *red* line. Because of the deployment of lockdown, which began in mid-April, the effective contact rate was reduced by a factor of 6.25.

With a similar explanation, the contact rate cut down for Gujarat after the lockdown was roughly 5.45 for a population of 2, 61, 838 million, according to the census for Gujarat [5]. Here, the growth rate shown by the purple line (denoting the actual data) is found to climb over the blue line (representing the modified model curve). This suggests that the curve is still rising even after the lockdown uplift. Thus, the effective contact rate had increased after uplifting the lockdown, which is visible by the rise of the actual data trend after the duration of 128 days from the start of the lockdown.

Delhi's effective contact rate shrinks by a factor of about 5.1 for the specified R_0 value 9.6. As per *Fig.* 6.6, the pace of the outbreak is very much similar to what was in Gujarat. However, the climb is not as sharp as in the case of Gujarat's curve and steadies soon. So, the actual growth trend (represented by the purple line) and blue line (the modified lockdown-based SIR prediction) meet near the end of the lockdown duration.

All the curvatures do not follow the high R_0 value of 9.6, according to which the entire mass population in any of the states is estimated to be infected by the 10th day of February. As an effect of lockdown imposition, the effective contact rate was reduced significantly, which helped to control the pandemic wave. However, the increase after the lockdown is still subtle in the growth pattern but much reduced from the original estimates. Apart from lockdown, an effective vaccination drive has also played a crucial role in tackling the growing infection. Given a large amount of initial infected population as a seed, the SIR estimation for the infected population during the second wave is significantly large as compared to the forecast for the first wave. The following section draws a parallel between the *alpha* and the *delta* variants in terms of their growth and how the lockdown period varies for the two waves.

6.3 Comparing the Two Waves of Covid-19

In this section, a comparative growth pattern analysis of both the first and second waves of Covid-19 has been done. It has already been inferred that the growth patterns of both waves follow an exponential trajectory following a logistic regression pattern. Table 6.1 depicts the parametric values *a, b, c, and d* with respect to Eq. 3.1 for the first wave. The same values are also calculated for the second wave 6.2.

Table 6.1 Estimated values of parameters for logistic fit for first wave

States	Estimated parameter values			
	a	b	c	d
Rajasthan	8.0991e+04	−1.1698e+03	3.1427e–02	1.5326e+02
Gujarat	1.0757e+05	−4.4275e+03	2.8945e–02	1.2263e+02
Maharashtra	3.4110e+06	−7.5880e+03	3.6533e–02	1.9026e+02
Delhi	2.3187e+05	3.7039e+02	6.4986e–02	1.2802e+02

Table 6.2 Estimated values of parameters for logistic fit for second wave

States	Logistic Parameter estimated values			
	a	b	c	d
Rajasthan	6.3341e+05	3.2076e+05	1.228e–01	3.110e+01
Gujarat	5.4022e+05	–2.848e+05	1.091e–01	2.830e+01
Maharashtra	–1.1946e+07	–1.1946e+07	0.8842e–02	–4.6524e+01
Delhi	8.0897e+05	6.270e+05	1.3268e–01	2.4312e+01

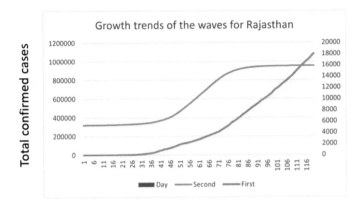

Fig. 6.7 A comparative analysis for the growth trends of first and second wave

From Tables 6.1 and 6.2, it is evident that in the case of the second variant, the parametric values range on a higher side which defines the sharp rise and curvature of the exponential curve. Comparatively higher values of *a, b, c, and d* in Table 6.2 thus indicate the more aggressive nature of Covid-19's second wave as compared to the first.

Figure 6.7 presents the growth rate of the two waves for the same duration of the consecutive years in which they hit. The figure shows the trend over the Rajasthan dataset from 3rd April, 2021 to 30th June, 2021 for the first wave and 3rd April, 2022 to 30th June, 2022 for the second wave, with the horizontal axis representing the days and vertical axis representing the number of infected persons. The initial growth pattern is steep in the case of the second wave (grey line) as compared to the first wave (yellow line), and it attains its peak very much earlier as compared to the *yellow* line. The *yellow* line was still peaking till the end of the graph. A similar trend can also be realized for the other three states as the growth dynamics are approximately the same for all the states.

Figure 6.8 defines the SIR model-based growth pattern of the disease. The first sub-figure shows a growth trend over the R_0 value of 6.0. On the other hand, the second sub-figure shows the growth trend of the disease for R_0 value = 9.6. In the second sub-figure, the peak attainment is quick and steep compared to the prior. Similarly, the spectrum for recovered people is also broad in sub-figure 2. Due to the

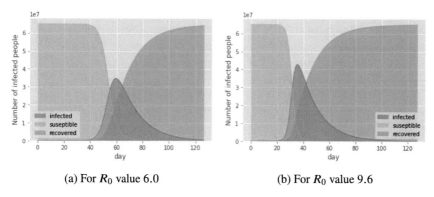

(a) For R_0 value 6.0   (b) For R_0 value 9.6

Fig. 6.8 SIR model-based growth dynamics of disease for R_0 value 6.0 and 9.6

Table 6.3 Predicting I_{max} based upon the R_0 values for first wave

State	Population count	R_0 value before lockdown	I_{max} estimate based on original R_0 value	R_0 value after lockdown	I_{max} estimate based on new R_0 value
Rajasthan	80 million [7]	6.0	78.80 million	6.0/4.175 = 1.437	76 million
Gujarat	65 million [5]	6.0	63.838 million	6.0/1.98 = 3.030	62.926 million
Maharashtra	124 million [6]	6.0	122.73 million	6.0/2.45 = 2.44	122.49 million
Delhi	30.2 million [3]	6.0	29.166 million	6.0/4.5 = 1.333	26.67 million

high R_0 value, for the second wave, the peak attained is also higher in comparison to the first wave. More people are likely to fetch infection with time as compared to the previous wave. This may be understood as an effect of a high seed infected population which was not there in the case of the first wave.

Comparing the lockdowns of the two phases, Tables 6.3 and 6.4 give an estimate of the total number of people to be infected for the given R_0 values based on Eq. 5.3 from Chap. 5.

Given the fact that the *Delta* variant is 60% more aggressive stain in comparison to the previous variant, the estimates for maximum infected people are pretty high. But interestingly, the total infected population for *Gujarat* and *Maharashtra* are on the lower end. The apparent reason is that the effective contact rate is far lower than the older stain. The lockdown has a significant impact in these two states in comparison to Rajasthan and Delhi, where the prediction of cases for the *Delta* variant is much more than the *Alpha* variant. But as seen earlier, the actual numbers differ due to rapid and large-scale vaccine drives that were carried out to reduce the *susceptible* population, which proved to be subtle. Moreover, many antibiotic drugs are now

Table 6.4 Predicting I_{max} based upon the R_0 values for second wave

State	Population count	R_0 value before lockdown	I_{max} estimate based on original R_0 value	R_0 value after lockdown	I_{max} estimate based on new R_0 value
Rajasthan	80 million [7]	9.6	79.20 million	9.6/6.1 = 1.573	76.29 million
Gujarat	65 million [5]	9.6	64.22 million	9.6/5.45 = 1.761	61.74 million
Maharashtra	124 million [6]	9.6	123.15 million	9.6/6.25= 1.536	119.93 million
Delhi	30.2 million [3]	9.6	29.50 million	9.6/5.1 = 1.882	27.52 million

available in the market, due to which the *recovery rate* also improves. These two aspects have been discussed in detail in the next section of this chapter. Due to these reasons, the actual numbers reflected in the data for the infected people per day as per [2] in comparison to the growth trends observed as per the SIR model are lower than what is being shown in the tables. But the variation does not mean that the I_{max} growth trend is meaningless. Only the numbers shown are not in accordance with the actual data. The growth pattern is correct, and hence, *Rajasthan* and *Delhi* had more infection rates than the previous wave.

However, the two variants have a vast difference in the mortality rate. The *Delta* variant is far more dangerous in comparison to the *Alpha* variant, given the fact that along with a high R_0 value, it has a high casualty rate as well. Figure 6.9 shows the trend of the growing deaths day-wise for all the four regions. The respective period of lockdowns for both the waves have been taken into consideration to analyse on the same grounds (considering the fact that infection reaches its peak during this time). In the figures, the *death toll* for the first wave is shown on the *left vertical axis*. For the second wave, the *right vertical axis* represents the same quantity. The *horizontal axis* of the graphs represents the *number of days*.

As per the observations from the graph, there is a huge difference in the rate of growth of the two curves, and the deaths that happened from the *Delta* variant are almost 20 to 30 times more in comparison to the casualties in the first wave. For Rajasthan, the number of people who died during the period of the first lockdown was nearly around 246 days, while the number of people who died during the second lockdown was 5, 601 [2]. For Gujarat, casualties during the first lockdown were 1280, while for the second wave, it drastically increased to 4, 688. Similarly, for Maharashtra , the respective values of death tolls are 3, 169 and 41, 202, and for Delhi, the values are 416 and 12, 708. Apart from Rajasthan, all the other states have a very high increase in the death rate for *Delta* variant, which is enough to convict the stain as more dangerous in comparison to the prior. However, strict lockdown procedures, vaccination, and effective drug treatment successfully controlled the

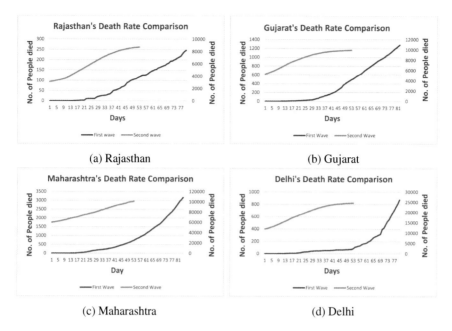

Fig. 6.9 Casualty graph trends for the two waves

upsurge, which is evident from the SIR model-based curve analysis. Despite the high R_0 value of the disease, the number of people fetching the infection was not that high, which certainly reduced the death numbers, which might have been even worse.

6.4 Vaccination Measures and Its Effect

Given the high pandemic destruction caused by the first wave of Covid-19, the vaccination drives and programs have been taken at utmost priority by the Indian government. Not only in India but throughout the world, the need for developing a successful vaccine as a precaution to *Corona*virus had been on the agenda of extremely high importance. As a result, a number of vaccines were developed namely *Pfizer, Covaxin, Covishield*, etc. [11]. In India, Covaxin and Covishield vaccines have been used, and both the vaccines have shown satisfactory results with the efficacy of 80% and 90% [9]. So, as per Eq. 5.4 from Chap. 5, Table 6.5 depicts the estimated vaccination that is required to be carried out considering the efficiency of the vaccine to be 80% effective.

The estimated population to be vaccinated is as per Table 6.5. Given this, the vaccination drives are also being carried out at a good rate. Figure 6.10 depicts the rate at which the vaccination has been carr0ied out across pan India [1]. Within a duration

Table 6.5 Prediction for population to be vaccinated

State	Population	Current R_0 value after lockdown	Predicted population to be vaccinated$((1 - \frac{1}{R_0}) *$ Population $* 0.8)$
Rajasthan	80 million [7]	1.573	23.31 million
Gujarat	65 million [5]	1.761	22.47 million
Maharashtra	124 million [6]	1.536	34.61 million
Delhi	30.2 million [3]	1.882	11.32 million

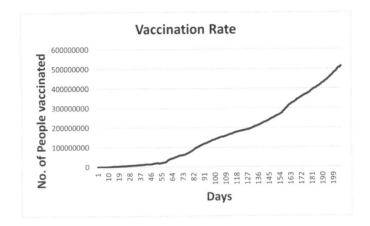

Fig. 6.10 Vaccination count curve for India

of 200 days, approximately 50×10^6 people were successfully vaccinated with the first dose of either *Covaxin, Covishield*, or *Sputnik*. This fast pace of vaccination reduces the number of susceptibles at an excellent rate which has helped to control the disease spread to a great extent.

Another factor that has played a massive role in deferring the pace of growth of the disease owing to its high contagion value is the fast recovery rate of the people. Figure 6.11 shows the recovery trend graphs for Rajasthan, Gujarat, Maharashtra, and Delhi. The steep jumps in the charts give a clear indication of the rapid pace at which the vaccination is carried out in the regions. As the number of infected people increases with the duration of the viral infection, more people enter the recovery phase. As per the trajectory of the SIR model, after a certain point, the growth rate function of infection moves in the reverse trajectory at the same rate, i.e. the curve of the recovery phase starts climbing, and the curve of infection rate starts dipping. The combined effect of vaccination and enhanced recovery rate of the individuals had cut down the number of *susceptibles* which acts as a feed to the infected phase. Since the number of people that may catch infection keeps reducing, the infection

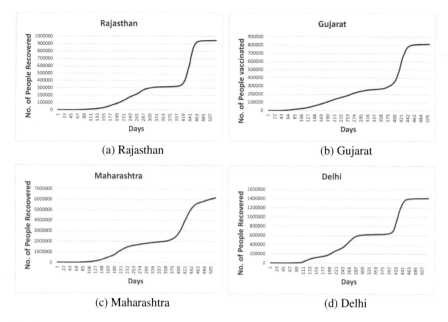

Fig. 6.11 Recovery trends

rate decreases. This happens due to the identification of suitable drugs, vaccination, etc.

On the other hand, since the infection phase has attained its maximum already, the number of people who can recover from the disease also increases and keeps increasing until the maximum possible population catches the infection. Thus, the factors like *lockdown*, *vaccination*, and *enhanced recovery rate* together play an important role in suppressing the devastating effect of the disease.

References

1. Covid-19 in India, Homepage: https://www.kaggle.com/datasets/sudalairajkumar/covid19-in-india?select=covid_vaccine_statewise.csv, Accessed on 24/03/2022
2. Covid-19 State-wise Time Series Data(till Sep'21), Homepage : https://www.kaggle.com/datasets/oddasparagus11/covid19-statewise-time-series-datatill-sep29, Accessed on 24/03/2022
3. Delhi Population, Homepage : http://www.populationu.com/in/delhi-population, Accessed on 24/03/2022
4. Delta Variant has 235% Higher Risk of ICU Admission than Original Virus. Medical News Today, 8 October 2021, Homepage: https://www.medicalnewstoday.com/articles/delta-variant-has-235-percent-higher-risk-of-icu-admission-than-original-virus, Accessed on 24/03/2022
5. Gujarat Population, Homepage : http://www.populationu.com/in/gujarat-population, Accessed on 24/03/2022

6. Maharashtra Population, Homepage : https://www.census2011.co.in/census/state/maharashtra.html, Accessed on 24/03/2022
7. Rajasthan Population, Homepage : http://www.populationu.com/in/rajasthan-population, Accessed on 24/03/2022
8. WHO Coronavirus (COVID-19) Dashboard, Homepage : https://covid19.who.int/, Accessed on 24/03/2022
9. Das, S., Kar, S.S., Samanta, S., Banerjee, J., Giri, B., Dash, S.K.: Immunogenic and reactogenic efficacy of covaxin and covishield: a comparative review. Immunol. Res. 1–27 (2022)
10. Hagen, A.: How dangerous is the delta variant (b. 1.617. 2). American Society of Microbiology (2021)
11. Sharma, K., Koirala, A., Nicolopoulos, K., Chiu, C., Wood, N., Britton, P.N.: Vaccines for covid-19: where do we stand in 2021? Paediatr. Respir. Rev. **39**, 22–31 (2021)
12. Sharma, N., Sharma, P., Basu, S., Bakshi, R., Gupta, E., Agarwal, R., Dushyant, K., Mundeja, N., Marak, Z., Singh, S. et al.: Second wave of the covid-19 pandemic in Delhi, India: high seroprevalence not a deterrent? Cureus **13**(10) (2021)
13. Shiehzadegan, S., Alaghemand, N., Fox, M., Venketaraman, V.: Analysis of the delta variant b. 1.617. 2 covid-19. Clinics Pract. **11**(4), 778–784 (2021)
14. Yang, W., Shaman, J.: Covid-19 pandemic dynamics in India and impact of the sars-cov-2 delta (b. 1.617. 2) variant (2021)

Chapter 7
Conclusions and Future Scope

This chapter concludes and summarizes the analysis presented in the book. Further, the possibilities of exploration of study in various aspects have also been discussed in brief.

7.1 Conclusions

The book's contents look into the current Covid-19 spread pattern, as determined by the SIR model based on the rise of Covid-19 in four key Indian regions. The book covers a variety of features of the disease's spread patterns for Covid-19 based on the SIR model. The study shows how the SIR model accurately predicts the development of real-time data. Despite the model's few assumptions, the model has the capabilities to validate a few critical facts. The model is also capable of making accurate predictions about the infection's growth rate-related parameters' increase and decrease. The experimental investigation of the real-time Covid-19 (first wave) data demonstrates this. One can uncover the reasons for deviations by bridging the gap between theoretical explanations and experimental outcomes. A similar analysis has been carried out to simulate the second wave dynamics in consonance with the SIR model establishments. Interestingly, the model brings out the peculiarities in the progression of the two Covid waves. Since both the waves follow an exponential rise in the initial phases, the jump in the rate of infection varies due to a big difference in the reproduction number R_0 values of the two diseases. This difference in the growth pattern of the disease has been justified on the basis of SIR model-based equations through graphical plots and visualizations. The reason along with high R_0 value for this variability is that the *Delta* variant has a high infection seed to the model in comparison to *Alpha* due to which both the range of infection as well as duration

R. Saxena et al., *Exploring Susceptible-Infectious-Recovered (SIR) Model for COVID-19 Investigation*, SpringerBriefs in Computational Intelligence, https://doi.org/10.1007/978-981-19-4175-7_7

of infection is high and acute. Based on these lines, the effect of lockdown on two waves has also been compared, and it has been observed that lockdown has played an important role during the second wave to keep the severity of the infection very much close to the first wave despite high infection rate of second Covid-19 wave.

In addition to the lockdown impact, timely vaccination drives and recovery rate improvement owing to proper treatment and therapies have played a significant role in improving the conditions in a very short period of time. This is evident from the fact that quickly after the release of the lockdown 2, the infection rate started dropping. In the current scenario, after a severe hit from *Delta* variant, another mutant named *Omicron* hit the nation near to the end of the year 2021. However, vaccination and the learnings from the past two waves did not allow the infection to create the sufferings in a similar manner. The casualty rate was far low in comparison to the previous two waves.

7.2 Future Scope

An exploration of this study can be carried out for the upcoming variants based on the model and for some other diseases which are not discussed in this book. Further, the study is focused about understanding the severity of the infection trend, its nature, etc. based on *Susceptible, Infected, and Recovery phases* (SIR) model. In order to make the predictions more accurate, the model needs to be fine-tuned by consideration of more factors like temperature conditions, average recovery rate, etc. which can give more power and flexibility to the model for accurate predictions. For this, the derived models of SIR like SEIR (*Susceptible, Exposed, Infected, and Recovery phases*) can be used. Also, the SIR model assumes that the same person can not be infected more than once by the disease (the infected cannot become susceptible again). However, for Covid-19, this is not true since there are multiple cases of disease re-occurrence. For this, SIS (*Susceptible, Infected, and Susceptible phases*) can be investigated.

Glossary

Epidemic The outburst of the disease to a mass in a very short period of time is referred to as *epidemic*.

Pandemic When an epidemic spreads across the globe, it is referred to as *pandemic*.

Coefficient of Determination (R^2) It is used to determine how differences in one variable may be explained by variations in another.

Transmission rate It is defined as the average number of persons infected each day by an infectious person.

Effective Contact rate (a) It is calculated by multiplying the transmission rate by the contact rate.

Recovery rate (b) It is defined as the recovery period (average number of days) taken by patient to recover from an infection.

Reproduction Number (R_0) It is defined as the ratio of *effective contact rate a* to *recovery rate b*. The value intuitively conveys how quickly the epidemic spreads.

Lockdown A lockdown is a policy that requires people or communities to remain in their current location owing to specific threats to themselves or others if they are allowed to travel and interact freely.

Herd Immunity When a significant section of a susceptible population gets immunised against a communicable disease, protecting the remainder of the population.

Vaccine Efficacy The relative reduction in cases among vaccinated people is measured by vaccination efficacy and effectiveness. When a study is conducted under ideal settings, such as during a clinical trial, vaccine efficacy is employed. When a trial is conducted in normal field (that is, less than precisely controlled) conditions, vaccine efficacy is utilised.

© The Author(s), under exclusive license to Springer Nature Singapore Pte Ltd. 2022   53
R. Saxena et al., *Exploring Susceptible-Infectious-Recovered (SIR) Model for COVID-19 Investigation*, SpringerBriefs in Computational Intelligence,
https://doi.org/10.1007/978-981-19-4175-7

Printed in the United States
by Baker & Taylor Publisher Services